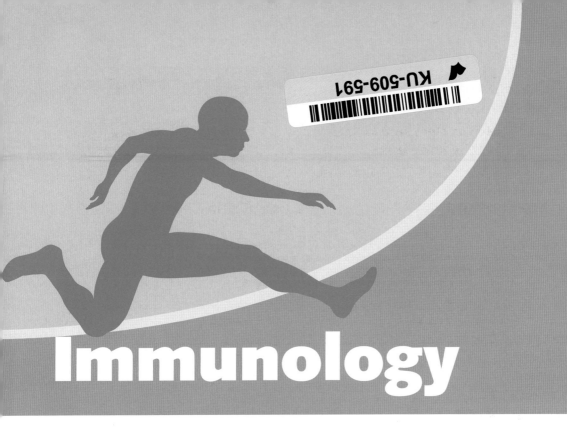

Immunology

Robert W. Novak, MD
Professor of Pathology
Northeastern Ohio Universities College of Medicine
Chair, Pathology and Laboratory Medicine
Akron Children's Hospital
Akron, Ohio

UK edition authors
James Griffin, Saimah Arif, and Arjmand Mufti

UK Series editor
Daniel Horton-Szar

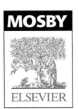

MOSBY

ELSEVIER

1600 John F. Kennedy Boulevard
Suite 1800
Philadelphia, PA 19103-2899

CRASH COURSE: IMMUNOLOGY   ISBN-13: 978-1-4160-3007-2
Copyright © 2006 by Mosby, Inc., an affiliate of Elsevier Inc.   ISBN-10: 1-4160-3007-7

Adapted from Crash Course Immunology and Haematology 2e by James Griffin, ISBN 0-7234-3246-5. © 2003, Elsevier Science Limited. All rights reserved.

The rights of James Griffin to be identified as the author of this work have been asserted by him in accordance with the Copyright Designs and Patents Act, 1988.

Library of Congress Cataloging-in-Publication Data

Immunology / Robert Novak ... [et al.].—1st ed.
    p. ; cm.—(Crash course)
    Includes bibliographical references and index.
    ISBN 1-4160-3007-7
    1. Immunology—Outlines, syllabi, etc.   2. Immunity—Outlines, syllabi, etc.
    [DNLM: 1. Immune System—physiology.   2. Immune System Diseases.   3. Immunity.
    QW 504 I363614 2006]   I. Novak, Robert, 1948-   II. Series.
    QR182.55.I47 2006
    616.07'9—dc22   2005054288

Commissioning Editor: Alex Stibbe
Developmental Editor: Stan Ward
Project Manager: David Saltzberg
Design: Andy Chapman
Cover Design: Antbits Illustration
Illustration Manager: Mick Ruddy

Printed in China.

Last digit is the print number:
9   8   7   6   5   4   3   2   1

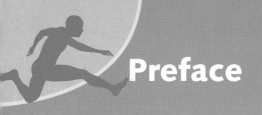

Preface

Immunology is an area of medical science in which constant progress in the understanding of both basic science and clinical practice is made on a daily basis. *Crash Course: Immunology* explains basic principles in detail so the reader can develop an understanding of the processes without being overly burdened by complexity. This text also introduces clinical concepts that carry forward into the clerkship year.

Robert W. Novak, MD

CRASH COURSE

Im

Other Titles in the Crash Course Series

There are 23 books in the Crash Course series in two ranges: Basic Science and Clinical. Each book follows the same format, with concise text, clear illustrations, and helpful learning features, including access online USMLE test questions.

Basic Science titles
Pathology
Nervous System
Renal and Urinary Systems
Gastrointestinal System
Respiratory System
Endocrine and Reproductive Systems
Metabolism and Nutrition
Pharmacology
Immunology
Musculoskeletal System
Cardiovascular System

Forthcoming:
Cell Biology and Genetics
Anatomy

Clinical titles
Surgery
Cardiology
History and Examination
Internal Medicine
Neurology
Gastroenterology

Forthcoming:
OBGYN
Psychiatry
Imaging
Pediatrics

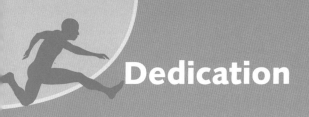

Dedication

*To
my associates, who provided me
the time to complete this project, and
to my family, Pamela and Marnie,
who understood.*

Contents

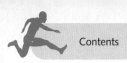

PRINCIPLES OF IMMUNOLOGY

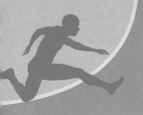

1. An Overview of Immunity

The human immune system has developed to protect the individual from the many and varied pathogens constantly present in the environment. It has two major divisions that are interlocking and complementary, the innate and adaptive immune systems.

Immunity is a state of relative resistance to disease.

Innate immune system

The innate immune system consists of physical and chemical barriers, cells and molecules that recognize a limited number of pathogen-associated molecular patterns, and effecter systems that facilitate destruction of pathogens. The receptors and effecters are fully defined in germ-line DNA and are always available. The innate immune response is rapid and invariant; there is no memory function or optimization as the reaction proceeds. Elements of the innate immune systems are essential to initiation of the response of the adaptive immune system, and innate effecters also function in the adaptive response.

Adaptive immune system

The adaptive immune system is centered about lymphocytes, which display a unique receptor that is generated through a process of clonal selection and expansion. There are two major classes of lymphocytes:

- B cells, which produce immunoglobulins, or molecules with a unique sequence that can combine with and destroy or neutralize pathogens or toxins.
- T cells, which collaborate with B cells and can also directly recognize and destroy pathogens and infected cells.

The adaptive immune system requires time to react initially, but it does possess a memory function that allows a more rapid and optimized response when a previously recognized threat is encountered. The number of antigens that the adaptive immune system recognizes is immense, but the recognition sites are a result of somatic DNA recombination and are not passed on to the next generation.

An **antigen** is any molecule that can be recognized by the adaptive immune system.
An **immunogen** is an antigen that evokes an immune response. Not all antigens are immunogens.
Epitopes are the small parts of the antigen recognized by the immune system. A single antigen can have more than one epitope, each of which is recognized by a different antibody or T-cell receptor (TCR).

Cellular and humoral elements of the innate and adaptive immune system are summarized in Fig. 1.1.

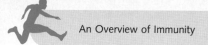

Components of the innate and adaptive immune systems		
	Innate system	Adaptive system
Cellular components	Monocytes/macrophages Neutrophils Eosinophils Basophils Mast cells Natural killer cells	B cells/Plasma cells T cells
Humoral components	Complement Cytokines Lysozyme Acute phase proteins Interferons	Antibody Cytokines

Fig. 1.1 Components of the innate and adaptive immune systems.

- Explain the main differences between innate and adaptive immunity.
- List the two major classes of lymphocytes.
- Explain the differences between antigen, immunogen, and epitope.
- List the main cellular and humoral components of the innate immune system.
- List the main cellular and humoral components of the adaptive immune system.

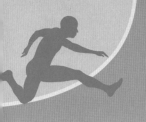

2. Sources of Cells of the Innate and Adaptive Immune Systems

Hematopoiesis is the formation and development of blood cells. This process depends upon stem cells, which divide to leave both a reserve population and cells committed to differentiating into the various blood cell lines. Differentiation occurs along one of three lineages:

1. Erythroid → erythrocytes.
2. Lymphoid → B and T lymphocytes and natural killer (NK) cells.
3. Myeloid → neutrophils, basophils, eosinophils, monocytes, and megakaryocytes.

The lymphoid and myeloid lines provide the cells of the immune system.

Sites of hematopoiesis

The main site of hematopoiesis changes during fetal development and maturation:

- Conception to 6 weeks: fetal yolk sac.
- 6 weeks to 6 months: fetal liver and spleen.
- 6 months onward: bone marrow.

Progenitor cells

In vitro hematopoiesis progenitors are detected via assays that identify cells capable of producing colonies (a colony-forming unit [CFU]). Granulocytes, erythrocytes, monocytes, and megakaryocytes are produced from a precursor known as CFU-GEMM. This precursor divides into an erythroid progenitor (CFU-E), a megakaryocyte precursor, an eosinophil precursor, and a granulocyte/monocyte precursor (CFU-GM). Lymphoid precursors become B cells or NK cells in the bone marrow or travel to the thymus, where they develop into T cells.

Growth factors

Cytokines and other growth factors regulate hematopoiesis. These factors are glycoproteins produced in the bone marrow, liver, and kidneys. Binding of the growth factor to surface receptors can trigger replication, differentiation, or functional activation, or it can inhibit apoptosis. Following stimulation by interferon-1 or tumor necrosis factor (TNF), stromal cells in the bone marrow produce many growth factors. Several growth factors, known as colony-stimulating factors (CSFs), have been identified:

- Multilineage CSF (IL-3): acts early in hematopoiesis to induce nonlymphoid cell production.
- Granulocyte–macrophage CSF: acts later on the same cells.
- Macrophage CSF and granulocyte CSF: are involved later still to produce monocytes and neutrophils.

An overview of hematopoiesis is presented in Fig. 2.1.

Growth factors are important in the maintenance of the bone marrow. Some are mainly homeostatic, providing feedback to maintain numbers of cells (e.g., erythropoietin), and some control response to immune reactions (e.g., interleukin-1 [IL-1]). Growth factors are summarized in Fig. 2.2.

Cytokines

Cytokines are soluble molecules secreted by one group of cells that mediate a variety of effects on other cells. When cells are acted upon by multiple cytokines simultaneously, the cytokines can have an additive, complementary, or antagonistic effect. Cytokines are commonly called interleukins (ILs), interferons (IFNs), tumor necrosis factors (TNFs), or colony-stimulating factors (CSFs). Cytokines can be divided into a number of categories by their function:

- Cytokines that promote hematopoiesis (outlined in the discussion of hematopoiesis; see Fig. 2.2).
- Cytokines that facilitate the innate immune response (Fig. 2.3).

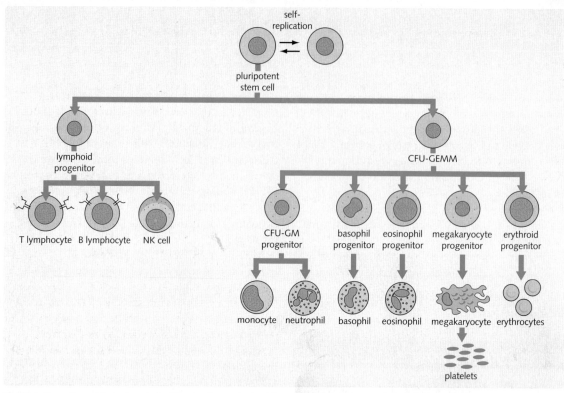

Fig. 2.1 Overview of hematopoiesis. Blood cells are derived from pluripotent stem cells usually found in the bone marrow. Exposure to different growth factors promotes the development of the different cell lines (CFU-GEMM, granulocyte, erythrocyte, monocyte, megakaryocyte colony-forming unit; CFU-GM, granulocyte-macrophage colony-forming unit; NK, natural killer).

Hematopoietic growth factors	
Factor	**Site of action**
Stem-cell factor	Pluripotent cells
IL-3	CFU-GEMM
GM-CSF	CFU-GM
G-CSF	Granulocyte precursor
M-CSF	Monocyte precursor
IL-5	Eosinophil progenitors
Erythropoietin	Erythrocyte progenitors
Thrombopoietin	Megakaryocyte progenitors
IL-6	B cell precursors
IL-2	T cell precursors
IL-1 and TNF	Stromal cells

Fig. 2.2 Growth factors in hematopoiesis (CFU-GEMM, granulocyte, erythrocyte, monocyte, megakaryocyte colony-forming unit; CFU-GM, granulocyte-monocyte colony-forming unit; GM-CSF, granulocyte-macrophage colony-stimulating factor, TNF, tumor necrosis factor).

- Cytokines that regulate adaptive immunity (Fig. 2.4).
- Cytokines that affect blood leukocyte movement and migration (Fig. 2.5).

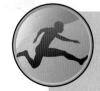 Cytokines are soluble molecules that mediate effects on other cells and activate and modulate the immune system.

Cytokine receptors

As can be seen in the outline of cytokines above, many cytokines have similar and overlapping activities. This is due in part to the limited number of families of cytokine receptors:

- Immunoglobulin superfamily receptors.
- Class I cytokine receptors.
- Class II cytokine receptors.
- TNF receptors.
- Chemokine receptors.

Cytokines that facilitate the innate immune response		
Cytokine	Source	Activity
IL-1	Monocytes Macrophages	Systemic inflammatory effect, including fever, acute-phase protein synthesis, T-cell activation
IL-6	T cells Other cells	Stimulates other T cells to produce IL-2, B cells to produce immunoglobulins, and stem cells
IFN-α IFN-β	Viral-infected cells	Interferes with viral replication, induces MHC class I expression
IFN-γ	Th1 cells	Activates NK cells and macrophages, induces MHC class II expression
TNF-α	Macrophages	Activates endothelial cells, vascular permeability

Fig. 2.3 Cytokines that facilitate the innate immune response (IL, interleukin; IFN, interferon; MHC, major histocompatibility complex; NK, natural killer; TNF, tumor necrosis factor).

Cytokines that regulate adaptive immunity		
Cytokine	Source	Activity
IL-2	Th1 cells	T cell growth factor
IL-4	Th2 cells	B cell growth factor
IL-5	T cells	B cell growth and immunoglobulin synthesis
IL-7	Marrow/thymic stromal cells	Pre-B and pre-T cell growth factor
IL-9	T cells	Activates mast cells
IL-10	Th2 cells and macrophages	Inhibits Th1 and macrophage function
IL-12	B cells and macrophages	Activates NK cells, Th1 proliferation
TNF-β	T cells	Killing by cytotoxic CD8 cells

Fig. 2.4 Cytokines that regulate adaptive immunity (IL, interleukin; NK, natural killer; TNF, tumor necrosis factor).

The limited number of cytokine receptors accounts for the overlapping function of the cytokines.

Cytokines that affect blood leukocyte movement and migration		
Cytokine	Source	Activity
IL-8	Monocyte Macrophages	Activates neutrophils, chemoattractant for neutrophils
RANTES	T cells Endothelial cells	Chemoattractant for monocytes, NK cells, eosinophils
Monocyte inflammatory proteins	Monocytes, T cells	Chemoattractant for monocytes, NK cells

Fig. 2.5 Cytokines that affect blood leukocyte movement and migration (IL, interleukin; RANTES, regulated on activation, T-cell expressed and secreted).

Class I chemokine receptors are by far the most common type of cytokine receptor. They consist of multiple subunits (dimers and trimers) with one subunit responsible for binding to the cytokine and another responsible for acting as the transmembrane signal transducer. Many class I cytokine receptors have a common signal-transducing unit (common γ chain), which probably accounts for the similarity of cellular responses to several cytokines. The correspondence of common cytokines and their receptors is shown in Fig. 2.6.

Cytokine-induced injury

Trauma, burns, and septic shock can induce massive cytokine release that can cause severe vascular leakage and organ damage, referred to as the systemic inflammatory reaction syndrome (SIRS). Many studies have shown that markedly elevated levels of TNF-α are associated with an unfavorable outcome in sepsis and trauma. Suppression of the cytokine response beyond a certain point appears to be desirable in the context of modern medical care. Since cytokines have a unique structure that allows them to interact with specific receptors, it is possible to produce antibodies to them in animals, which can then be fused with mouse myeloma cells to produce monoclonal antibodies in cell culture. A number of monoclonal antibodies that act to inhibit the function or increase the clearance of cytokines, especially TNF-α, have been used to try to improve outcomes in sepsis or to control severe prolonged inflammatory reactions, such as those observed in autoimmune conditions.

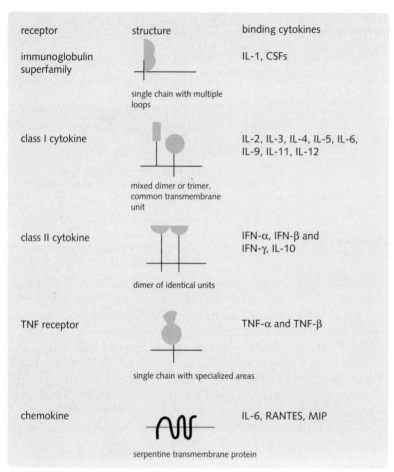

Fig. 2.6 Common cytokines and their receptors (IL, interleukin; IFN, interferon; CSF, colony-stimulating factor; TNF, tumor necrosis factor; RANTES, regulated on activation, T-cell expressed and secreted; MIP, macrophage inflammatory protein).

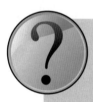

- List the three lineages into which stem cells differentiate.
- Summarize changes in the site of hematopoiesis during fetal growth and maturation.
- Define colony-forming unit.
- List three colony-stimulating factors.
- Define cytokines. Summarize their effect on the immune system.
- List the families of cytokine receptors. Identify the most common.
- Define SIRS.

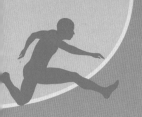

3. The Innate Immune System

Innate defenses can be classified into three main groups:
1. Barriers to infection.
2. Cells.
3. Serum proteins and the complement system.

Barriers to infection

Physical and mechanical
Skin and mucosal membranes act as physical barriers to the entry of pathogens. Tight junctions between cells prevent the majority of pathogens from entering the body. The flushing actions of tears, saliva, and urine protect epithelial surfaces from colonization. High oxygen tension in the lungs and body temperature can also inhibit microbial growth.

In the respiratory tract, mucus is secreted to trap microorganisms. They are then mechanically expelled by:
• Beating cilia (mucociliary escalator).
• Coughing.
• Sneezing.

Chemical
The growth of microorganisms is inhibited at acidic pH (e.g., in the stomach and vagina). Lactic acid and fatty acids in sebum (produced by sebaceous glands) maintain the skin pH between 3 and 5. Enzymes such as lysozyme (found in saliva, sweat, and tears) and pepsin (present in the gut) destroy microorganisms.

Biologic (normal flora)
A person's normal flora are formed when nonpathogenic bacteria colonize epithelial surfaces. Normal flora protect the host by:
• Competing with pathogenic bacteria for nutrients and attachment sites.
• Production of antibacterial substances.

The use of antibiotics disrupts the normal flora, and pathogenic bacteria are then more likely to cause disease.

Cells of the innate immune system

Monocytes
Appearance and structure
Monocytes (Fig. 3.1) tend to be the largest circulating blood cell, up to 25 μm in diameter. They have a large, kidney-shaped nucleus. Nucleoli are often present, giving the nucleus a "moth-eaten" appearance. The cytoplasm contains many lysosomes and vacuole-like spaces that produce a "ground-glass" appearance. Microtubules, microfilaments, pinocytotic vesicles, and filopodia or pseudopodia are present around the edge of the cell.

Location
Monocytes spend only a few days in the blood before migrating into the tissues, where they differentiate to become macrophages. Macrophages survive for several months to years in connective tissue.

Function
Mononuclear phagocytes are the key cells for initiation of both the innate and adaptive immune response. Monocytes and macrophages express on

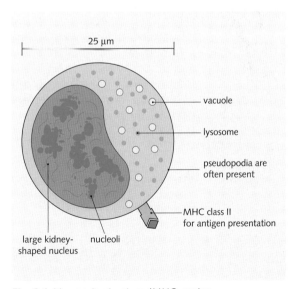

Fig. 3.1 Monocyte structure (MHC, major histocompatibility complex).

their surface receptors called Toll-like receptors (TLR). These receptor molecules often operate in pairs and are attached to an intracellular signaling complex of four molecules (MyD88, Mal, Tram, and Trif), which can activate kinases and lead to phosphorylation of transcription factors that mediate the production of cytokines that induce inflammation (the primary activity of the innate immune system) and also initiate T- and B-cell activation (an important event of the adaptive immune response). There are 10 known TLR; the known associations with specific pathogens are presented in Fig. 3.2.

Known associations of TLR with specific pathogens	
TLR	**Pathogen molecular pattern**
TLR 1 and 2	Bacterial lipopeptides of gram-positive bacteria, mycobacteria, and parasites
TLR 2 and 6	Lipoteichoic acid of gram-positive bacteria and zymosan of fungi
TLR 3	Double-stranded viral DNA
TLR 4	Lipopolysaccharide of gram-negative bacteria
TLR 5	Flagellin of motile bacterial
TLR 7 and 8	Single-stranded viral DNA
TLR 9	DNA CpG motifs present in DNA viruses and some bacteria

Fig. 3.2 Known associations of TLR with specific pathogens (TLR, Toll-like receptors).

The mononuclear phagocytes also ingest pathogens and foreign materials, break them down, and then present antigen fragments on their surfaces complexed with other proteins, acting as antigen-presenting cells (APC), another important element in the initiation of the adaptive immune response. A summary of the key role that mononuclear phagocytes play in the immune response is illustrated in Fig. 3.3.

Neutrophils

Neutrophils (Fig. 3.4), also known as polymorphonuclear leukocytes, measure 9–15 µm in diameter. They have distinctive nuclei containing 2–5 lobes connected by thin chromatin threads. In females, the nucleus has a "drumstick" appendage that contains the inactivated X chromosome. Neutrophils have few mitochondria and large stores of glycogen. The cytoplasm contains an abundance of three types of granule:

1. Small, specific granules (0.1 µm in diameter) containing antimicrobial enzymes and other agents.
2. Azurophilic granules (0.5 mm in diameter) similar to lysosomes.
3. Tertiary granules containing gelatinase, cathepsins, and glycoproteins.

Location

Neutrophils circulate in blood for up to 10 hours. In response to chemotactic agents, they migrate into tissues, where they survive for 1–3 days.

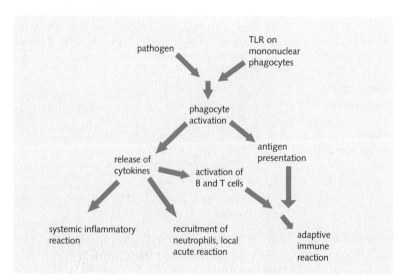

Fig. 3.3 Overview of the role of mononuclear phagocytes in immune response.

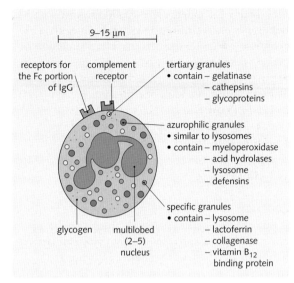

Fig. 3.4 Neutrophil structure.

Within the Fig. 3.4 diagram:

9–15 µm

receptors for the Fc portion of IgG

complement receptor

tertiary granules
• contain – gelatinase
– cathepsins
– glycoproteins

azurophilic granules
• similar to lysosomes
• contain – myeloperoxidase
– acid hydrolases
– lysosome
– defensins

specific granules
• contain – lysosome
– lactoferrin
– collagenase
– vitamin B$_{12}$ binding protein

glycogen

multilobed (2–5) nucleus

Function

Neutrophils are the first cells to reach sites of inflammation, and, once defunct, they are the major constituent of pus. They destroy microorganisms by phagocytosis and release of hydrolytic enzymes.

Killing by neutrophils

The process of phagocytosis allows cells to engulf matter that needs to be destroyed. The cell can then digest the material in a controlled fashion before releasing the contents. The process of phagocytosis is shown in Fig. 3.5.

Microbial degradation within the phagolysosome occurs along two pathways: one requires oxygen; the other is oxygen independent.

Oxygen-independent degradation

Neutrophil granules contain several antimicrobial agents, including:

• Lysozyme (splits peptidoglycan).
• Lactoferrin and reactive nitrogen intermediates (which complex with, and deprive pathogens of, iron).
• Proteolytic enzymes (degrade dead microbes).
• Defensins, cathepsin G, and cationic proteins (damage microbial membranes).

Oxygen-dependent degradation

A respiratory burst, increased oxygen consumption, accompanies oxygen-dependent degradation. Granule oxidases, along with NADPH and NADPH oxidase, reduce molecular oxygen to superoxide radicals ($O_2^{\bullet-}$), a reactive oxygen species. The

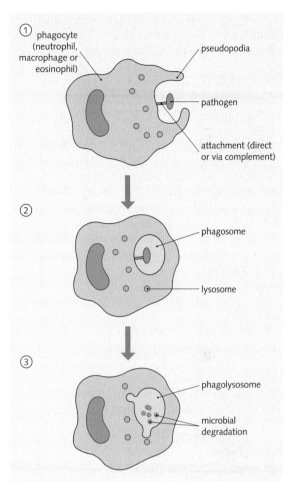

Fig. 3.5 Phagocytosis. Phagocytes sense an organism and bind it via nonspecific receptors or via complement or antibody. Pseudopodia extend from the surface of the cell to surround the pathogen (1). The pseudopodia fuse around the organism, producing a vesicle known as a phagosome (2). Lysosomes fuse with the phagosome to form phagolysosomes (3). Chemicals within the lysosome and other granules that fuse with the phagolysosome lead to degradation of the organism. The microbial products are then released.

Within Fig. 3.5 diagram:

① phagocyte (neutrophil, macrophage or eosinophil)

pseudopodia

pathogen

attachment (direct or via complement)

② phagosome

lysosome

③ phagolysosome

microbial degradation

following reactions also occur, producing other reactive species:

$$2O_2^{\bullet-} + 2H^+ \rightarrow H_2O_2 + O_2$$
$$O_2^{\bullet-} + H_2O_2 \rightarrow OH^{\bullet} + OH^- + O_2$$
$$H_2O_2 + Cl^- \rightarrow OCl^- + H_2O$$
(catalyzed by myeloperoxidase)
$$OCl^- + amine \rightarrow chloramines$$

Hypochlorus acid (HOCl) and chloramines live longer than the other oxidizing agents and are probably the most important target-killing compounds *in vivo*. If a target cannot be easily phagocytosed, there may be extracellular release of granule contents, causing tissue damage.

Eosinophils
Appearance and structure
Eosinophils (Fig. 3.6) are similar to neutrophils but larger: 12–17 µm in diameter. Their nucleus is sausage shaped and usually bilobed. They have a small, central Golgi apparatus and limited rough endoplasmic reticulum and mitochondria. Eosinophils contain large, ovoid, specific granules and azurophilic granules. The specific granules (1–1.5 µm long) have a crystalloid center containing major basic protein, eosinophilic cationic protein, and eosinophil-derived neurotoxin. The outside of the granule contains several enzymes, including histaminase, peroxidase, and cathepsin.

Location
They are primarily found in the tissues, spending less than 1 hour in blood.

Function
Their primary function is to combat parasitic infection. Eosinophils also phagocytose antigen–antibody complexes.

Basophils
Appearance and structure
Basophils (Fig. 3.7) are 14–16 µm in diameter with a bilobed "S-shaped" nucleus. They are named after their highly basophilic cytoplasmic specific granules but also contain azurophilic granules. Specific granules (0.5 µm in diameter) are large, membrane-bound round or oval structures. They push into the plasma membrane, causing a "roughened perimeter." The granules contain heparin, histamine, chemotactic factors, and peroxidase.

Location
The life span is unknown; however, they survive for 1–2 years in mice.

Function
It is not clear whether basophils are the precursors to mast cells, with which they share many similarities. Basophils are thought to mediate inflammatory responses.

Natural killer (NK) cells
NK cells are non-T, non-B cells of lymphoid lineage. They are also known as large granular lymphocytes and comprise 5–10% of circulating lymphocytes. NK cells are primarily involved in killing tumors and cells infected with intracellular pathogen, primarily viruses, *Leishmania* and *Listeria monocytogenes*. NK cells are nonspecifically activated by mitogens and the interferons, IL-2 and IL-12. NK cells are known as lymphokine-activated killer cells, because activation by IL-2, a lymphokine (produced by lymphoid cells), results in increased "killing" ability.

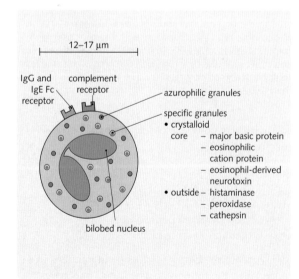

Fig. 3.6 Eosinophil structure.

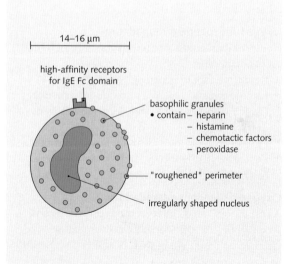

Fig. 3.7 Basophil structure.

Appearance and structure

NK cells are a subset of circulating lymphocytes. They are generally larger than B and T cells and have granules in the cytoplasm, as illustrated in Fig. 3.8.

Function

NK cells utilize cell-surface receptors to identify virally modified or cancerous cells. One set of receptors activates NK cells, initiating killing; others inhibit the cells:

- Activating receptors include calcium-binding C-lectins, which recognize certain cell-surface carbohydrates. Because these carbohydrates are present on the surface of normal host cells, a system of inhibitory receptors acts to prevent killing.
- Killer inhibitor receptors (KIRs), members of the immunoglobulin gene superfamily, are specific for class I MHC molecules. Human NK cells also express an inhibitory receptor (a heterodimer CD94:NKG2) that detects nonclassic class I molecules.

Virally infected cells often express reduced levels of MHC class I or, along with some tumor cells, altered class I MHC molecules. A reduction in MHC class I molecules avoids killing by cytotoxic CD8$^+$ T cells but makes the cells susceptible to lysis by NK cells.

NK cells can also destroy antibody-coated target cells, regardless of the presence of MHC molecules, a process known as antibody-dependent cell-mediated cytotoxicity. This occurs because killing is initiated by cross-linking of receptors for the Fc portion of IgG1 and IgG3.

NK cells are not clonally restricted, have no memory, and are not very specific in their action. They induce apoptosis in target cells (Fig. 3.9) by:

- Ligation of Fas or TNF receptors on the target cells (NK cells produce TNF and exhibit FasL). This initiates a sequence of caspase recruitment and activation, resulting in apoptosis.
- Degranulation by NK cells, which releases perforins and granzymes. Perforin molecules

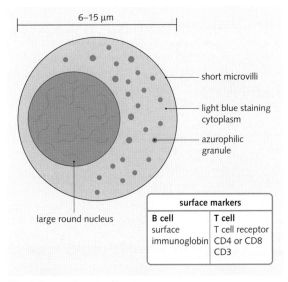

Fig. 3.8 Lymphocyte structure.

6–15 μm

short microvilli

light blue staining cytoplasm

azurophilic granule

large round nucleus

surface markers	
B cell	**T cell**
surface immunoglobin	T cell receptor
	CD4 or CD8
	CD3

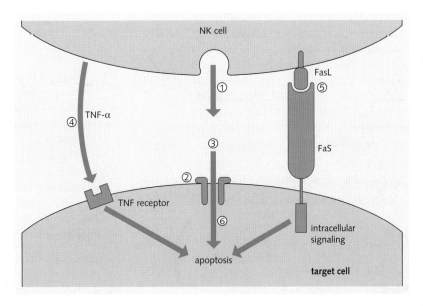

Fig. 3.9 Mechanisms of killing by natural killer (NK) cells (1). Activation of NK cells in the absence of an inhibitory signal results in degranulation (2). Perforins form a pore in the target cell, allowing entry of granzymes (3). TNF produced by NK cells acts on the target's cell receptors (4). FasL interacts with target cell Fas (5). Intracellular signaling from Fas, TNF receptors, and granzymes results in apoptosis (6).

NK cell

FasL

⑤

①

TNF-α

④

③

FaS

②

TNF receptor

⑥

intracellular signaling

apoptosis

target cell

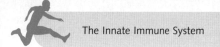

insert into and polymerize within the target cell membrane. This forms a pore through which granzymes can pass. Granzyme B then initiates apoptosis from within the target cell cytoplasm.

Soluble proteins of the innate immune system

The soluble proteins that contribute to innate immunity can be divided into antimicrobial serum agents, proteins produced by cells, and a series of proenzymes that constitute the complement system.

Antimicrobial serum agents are also called acute-phase proteins because they increase rapidly after activation of the innate immune response. The major antimicrobial serum agents include the following:

- Lactoferrin: iron-binding protein that competes with pathogens for iron, an essential metabolite.
- C-reactive protein (CRP): binds to C-polysaccharide cell component of bacteria and fungi and activates complement via the classic pathway.
- Mannan-binding lectin (MBL): binds to bacterial cell wall polysaccharides and activates complement via the lectin pathway.
- Serum amyloid A protein (SAP): binds to bacterial cell wall lipopolysaccharide and serves as a receptor for phagocyte attachment.

Interferons are the major proteins that are produced by virally infected cells. The alpha and beta interferons are produced by virally infected cells, and they induce a state of viral resistance in adjacent cells by inducing genes that produce products that destroy viral DNA and induce MHC class I expression. Interferon gamma is produced by activated NK cells, and it recruits NK cells and macrophages.

The complement system

The complement system consists of over 20 serum glycoproteins, synthesized principally by hepatocytes. The complement system is important for the recruitment of inflammatory cells and the killing or opsonization of pathogens.

Many of the complement components circulate in the serum as proenzymes (functionally inactive enzymes) that require proteolytic cleavage for activation. The larger fragment binds to the surface of the substrate, and the smaller one diffuses away. Once a component is activated, it catalyses the next step of the pathway. Components remain in the activated state for only a short time.

There are three pathways of complement activation—classic, lectin, and alternative pathways—that terminate in a common final pathway. An overview of the complement system is given in Fig. 3.10.

The classic pathway
Antibodies (particularly IgG and IgM), bound to antigen, can activate the classical pathway via their CH2 or CH3 domains. C1 (a complex of one C1q and two C1s and C1r molecules) binds to immunoglobulin via the C1q component. This results in:

- Activation of C1r and C1s.
- C1s activation of C4, which then binds C2.
- C2 activation by C1s.
- Formation of C3 convertase (the C4b/C2a complex).

The lectin pathway
Mannan-binding lectin, which is normally found in serum, binds to MBL-associated serine proteases (MASP). This complex bears structural homology to the C1 complex. When MBL binds to carbohydrate on the surface of bacteria, MASP is activated. MASP then acts on C4 and C2 to generate the C3 convertase of the classic pathway.

The alternative pathway
C3 contains a labile thioester bond that is susceptible to spontaneous hydrolysis. C3b, generated in this way, is deposited on host and microbial surfaces. Certain features of microbial surfaces allow persistence of C3b:

- Lack of inactivating regulatory molecules (present on eukaryotic cell membranes).
- On microbial surfaces, there is an inreased tendency of C3b to bind factor B, rather than factor H (an inhibitory molecule).

Activation of factor B by factor D results in the formation of C3bBb, which is a C3 convertase.

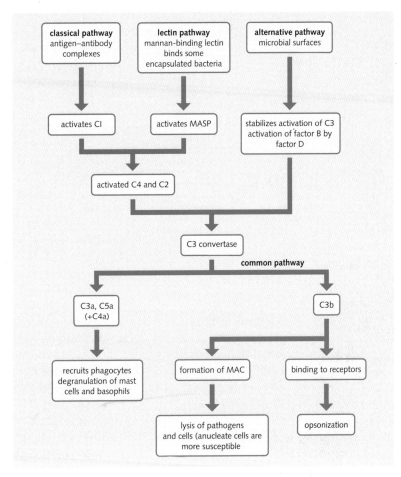

Fig. 3.10 Overview of the complement system. Cell lysis by complement is due to formation of the membrane attack complex (MAC). This is formed when C5b, C6, C7, C8, and C9 bind together to form a 10-nm pore in the cell surface (MASP, Mannan-binding lectin–associated serine protease).

The common terminal pathway

C5 convertase is formed from C3 convertase and C3b. Because C3 convertase is able to produce large quantities of C3b, it acts as a major amplification step in the complement pathway. Cleavage of C5 produces activated C5b, which sequentially binds C6, C7, and C8. C5b67 inserts into the cell membrane, and C8 binds to this membrane-bound complex. Between 10 and 16 molecules of C9, a perforin-like molecule, bind to the C5b678 complex to create an ion-permeable pore. The C5b6789 complex, which is also called the membrane attack complex (MAC), results in osmotic lysis of the cell.

Functions of complement

The products of the complement pathway play an important role in both adaptive and innate immunity (Fig. 3.11).

Inhibitors of complement

Inhibitors of the complement pathway are important in regulating its activity and preventing complement-mediated damage of healthy cells. Factors that inhibit complement include:
- Membrane cofactor protein, complement receptor type 1, C4b-binding protein and factor H, which prevent assembly of C3 convertase.
- Decay-accelerating factor, which accelerates decay of C3 convertase.
- C1 inhibitor, which inhibits C1.
- Factor I and membrane cofactor protein, which cleave C3b and C4b.
- CD59 (protectin), which prevents the formation of MAC.

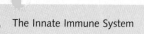
Functions of complement	
Function	**Notes**
Cell lysis	Insertion of MAC causes lysis of gram-negative bacteria. Nucleated cells are more resistant to lysis because they endocytose MAC
Inflammation	C3a, C4a, C5a cause degranulation of mast cells and basophils C3a and C5a are chemotactic for neutrophils
Opsonization	Phagocytes have C3b receptors, which means that they are able to phagocytose antigen coated in C3b
Solubilization and clearance of immune complexes	Complement prevents immune complex precipitation and solubilizes complexes that have already been precipitated. Complexes coated in C3b bind to CR1 on red blood cells. The complexes are then removed in the spleen

Fig. 3.11 Functions of complement (MAC, membrane attack complex).

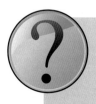

- What noncellular innate barriers provide a defense against infection?
- In what ways do cells of the innate immune system combat pathogens?
- Why is pathogen killing by phagocytes accompanied by a "respiratory burst"?
- What differences are seen between macrophages and neutrophils?
- How do NK cells identify virally infected and tumor cells for killing but do not kill normal cells?
- What are the complement cascade and the actions of complement?
- What is meant by the term "acute-phase response"? What proteins are involved?

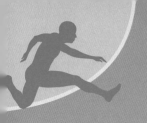

4. The Adaptive Immune System

Lymphocytes: cells of the adaptive immune system

Lymphocytes are produced in bone marrow and develop into fully functional B, T, and NK cells in lymphoid organs. Different functional classes of lymphocytes are not morphologically distinguishable (although most large granular lymphocytes are NK cells). Functional types of lymphocytes are distinguished by molecules that are expressed on their surfaces. These molecules are unique receptors and clusters of molecules that interact with the receptors or perform other functions that define the lymphocyte. The characteristic membrane-bound molecules (called cluster designations [CD]) are:

- B cells: B-cell receptor (BCR), CD-19, CD-20, CD-32, CD-40, and HLA-DR.
- T cells: T-cell receptor (TCR), CD2, CD3, CD4 (T helper cells) or CD8 (T suppressor/cytotoxic cells), CD7, and CD-28.
- NK cells: CD2, CD7, CD-16, CD-25, CD-56, and CD-57.

B-cell and T-cell receptors

The immunoglobulin domain

B-cell and T-cell surface receptors are members of the immunoglobulin gene superfamily. Genes in this family code for proteins composed of motifs called immunoglobulin domains. Members of this gene family include the following:

- Immunoglobulin (B-cell receptor).
- T-cell receptor.
- MHC molecules.
- T-cell accessory molecules such as CD4.
- Certain adhesion molecules (e.g., ICAM-1, ICAM-2, and VCAM-1).
- Poly-Ig receptor.
- Ig-α/Ig-β heterodimer.

Each domain is approximately 110 amino acids in length. The polypeptide chain in each domain is folded into seven or eight antiparallel beta strands.

The strands are arranged to form two opposing sheets, linked by a disulphide bond and hydrophobic interactions. This compact structure is called the immunoglobulin fold.

Structure of B-cell and T-cell surface antigen receptors
Structure of immunoglobulin

The B-cell surface receptor is a membrane-bound immunoglobulin (mIg) molecule. mIg recognizes the conformational structure (shape) of antigenic epitopes. Ig is composed of two light and two heavy chains. In the B-cell receptor (Fig. 4.1), mIg associates with two Ig-α/Ig-β dimers (members of the immunoglobulin gene superfamily). Signal transduction through the mIg is thought to be mediated by the Ig-α/Ig-β heterodimers.

Ig is also secreted by plasma cells. The extracellular portion of mIg is identical in structure to secretory Ig. mIg differs from secreted Ig (sIg) because it has transmembrane and cytoplasmic portions that anchor it to the membrane. Different Ig

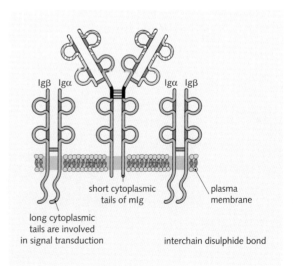

Fig. 4.1 Structure of the B-cell surface receptor. Membrane-bound immunoglobulin is nonsignaling. It associates with two Ig-α/Ig-β heterodimers (members of the immunoglobulin gene superfamily), which have long cytoplasmic domains capable of transducing a signal.

classes can be expressed on the same B cell and may indicate the stage of development of the B cell (e.g., a mature, but antigenically unchallenged, B cell expresses both mIgM and mIgD). The antigenic specificity of all of the mIg molecules expressed on any given B cell is the same.

The T-cell surface antigen receptor

Antigen recognition by T cells differs from antigen recognition by B cells:

- T cells recognize antigen only when it is associated with a molecule of the MHC.
- T cells recognize peptide fragments of an antigen in association with MHC molecules; it is not in original conformation. Therefore, antigen must be processed before it is presented to the T cell.

The T-cell surface antigen receptor consists of the T-cell receptor (TCR) associated with CD3. The TCR is a heterodimer, comprising α- and β-chains, or γ- and δ-chains. Approximately 95% of T cells express αβ-receptors. T cells expressing γδ-receptors are found particularly in epithelial tissues. The TCR is structurally similar to the immunoglobulin Fab region. Each chain consists of two immunoglobulin domains, one variable and one constant, linked by a disulphide bond. As in the variable domains of immunoglobulin, three variable regions on each chain combine to form the antigen-binding site.

CD3 is made up of three polypeptide dimers, consisting of four or five different peptide chains. The dimers are γε, δε, and ζζ (found in 90% of CD3 molecules) or ζη. The γ-, δ-, and ε-chains are members of the Ig gene superfamily. The TCR recognizes and binds antigen. CD3, functionally analogous to the Ig-α/Ig-β heterodimer in B cells, is involved in signal transduction (Fig. 4.2).

The major histocompatibility complex (MHC)

Major histocompatibility complex (MHC) is a generic term for a group of molecules produced by higher vertebrate species. The human leukocyte antigen (HLA) system is the human MHC.

The MHC is a cluster of tightly linked genes, found on the short arm of chromosome 6. Gene products of the MHC are involved in peptide binding, processing, and presentation. Several complement proteins (C4, C2, and factor B), cytokines (TNF-α), transcription factors, and enzymes are also encoded within the MHC. MHC molecules allow the immune system to detect self from nonself and to detect the presence of pathogens. T cells recognize antigen in the context of MHC molecules.

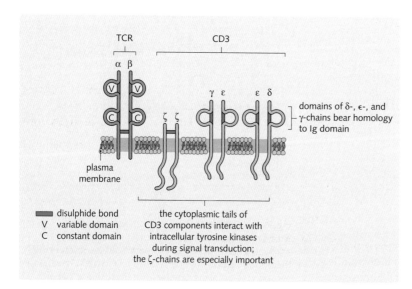

Fig. 4.2 Structure of the T-cell surface antigen receptor. Negative charges on the transmembrane portion of CD3 components interact with positive charges on the T-cell receptor (TCR). This maintains the complex. Antigen is detected by the TCR, but the signal is transduced by CD3.

The MHC genes

MHC genes exhibit a high degree of polymorphism; that is, they exhibit considerable diversity (there are more than 100 identified alleles for human leukocyte antigen B [HLA-B]). This means that most individuals will be heterozygous at most MHC loci and that any two randomly selected individuals are very unlikely to have identical HLA alleles. Diversity of the MHC increases the chance that a person will be able to mount an adaptive response against a pathogen. The genetic loci are tightly linked, so that a set is inherited from each parent. The genes are divided into three regions, each region encoding one of the three classes of the MHC; class I, class II, and class III (Fig. 4.3). The MHC alleles exhibit codominance, which means that both alleles are expressed.

 A complete set of MHC alleles inherited from one parent is referred to as a haplotype.

Structure and function of the MHC

Class I and class II MHC molecules are glycoproteins expressed on the cell surface and consist of cytoplasmic, transmembrane, and extracellular portions (Fig 4.4). Both class I and class II molecules exhibit broad specificity in their binding of peptide. The polymorphism of the MHC is largely concentrated in the peptide-binding cleft. A summary of the differences between class I and II MHC molecules is shown in Fig. 4.5.

MHC restriction

T cells are able to recognize antigen only in the context of self-MHC molecules (self-MHC restriction). CD8$^+$ T cells recognize antigen only in association with class I MHC molecules (class I MHC restricted). CD4$^+$ T cells recognize antigen only in association with class II MHC molecules (class II MHC restricted).

Antigen processing and presentation

MHC molecules do not present whole antigen. The antigen is degraded into peptide fragments before binding can occur. There are different pathways of antigen processing for class I and class II MHC. The pathways are summarized in Fig. 4.6.

Antigen-presenting cells (APCs) process and present antigen to CD4$^+$ T cells in association with class II molecules. These cells express high levels of class II MHC molecules. APCs include the following:
- Dendritic cells, including Langerhans' cells.
- Macrophages.
- B cells.

Structure and function of CD4 and CD8

CD4 and CD8 are "accessory" molecules that play an important role in the T cell–antigen interaction. CD4 and CD8 have two important functions:
- They bind MHC class II and class I molecules, respectively, thereby strengthening the T cell–antigen interaction.
- They function as signal transducers.

The role of CD4 and CD8 in antigen–receptor binding is shown in Fig. 4.7.

Genetic rearrangement in BCR and TCR formation

The large number of BCR and TCR specificities that can recognize antigens arises from a process of genetic recombination. The germ-line configurations

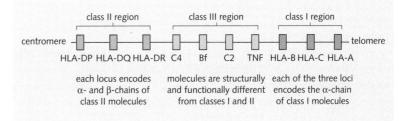

Fig. 4.3 Genetic organization of the human leukocyte antigen (HLA) complex. Only the classic genes are shown. The HLA complex is located in a 3–4 megabase sequence on the short arm of chromosome 6.

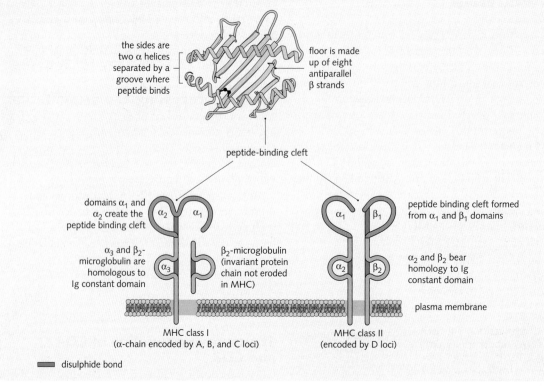

Fig. 4.4 Structure of class I and class II major histocompatibility complex molecules. The peptide-binding cleft of a class I molecule is also shown as seen from above.

Differences between class I and class II major histocompatibility complex molecules		
	Class I	**Class II**
Size of bound peptide	8–9 amino acids	13–18 amino acids (binding cleft more open)
Peptide from	Cytosolic antigen	Intravesicular or extracellular antigen
Expressed by	All nucleated cells, especially T cells, B cells, macrophages, other antigen-presenting cells, neutrophils	B cells, macrophages, other antigen-presenting cells, epithelial cells of the thymus, activated T cells
Recognized by	CD8+ T cells	CD4+ T cells

Fig. 4.5 Differences between class I and class II major histocompatibility complex molecules.

of BCR light chains and heavy chains and the TCR alpha, beta, delta, and gamma chains consist of groups of V (variable), D (diverse, BCR heavy chains and TCR beta and delta chains only), and J (joining) segments that recombine to generate a unique variable portion of the receptor during the antigen-independent development from a lymphocyte stem cell into a mature T or B cell. The chromosomal location of the segments in BCR and

TCR receptors and the number of functional V, D, and J segments in each germ-line region are presented in Fig. 4.8.

BCR rearrangements

BCR rearrangements occur in a specific sequence. Heavy-chain rearrangement occurs first in the pro (DJ-rearranged) B cell and pre (VDJ-rearranged) B cell. This process is illustrated in Fig. 4.9.

Fig. 4.6 Routes of antigen processing. A. Class I molecules present endogenous antigens. Cytosolic antigen is degraded by proteosomes and transported into the rough endoplasmic reticulum (ER), where peptides are loaded onto class I molecules. The MHC-peptide complex is transported via the Golgi apparatus to the cell surface. B. Class II molecules present exogenous antigens that have been phagocytosed or endocytosed into intracellular vesicles. The MHC molecule is transported from the rough ER to the vesicle by the invariant chain (Ii). It is displaced from the MHC molecule by processed antigen, which is then presented at the cell surface (MHC, major histocompatibility complex).

A
class I (endogenous) presentation

B
class II (exogenous) presentation

cell surface

antigen internalized by phagocytosis or endocytosis

MHC: antigen complex

early endosome

transport vesicle

degraded antigen

class II storage vesicle

Golgi apparatus

MHC: antigen complex

invariant chain

peptides

antigen

rough ER

proteosome

ribosome

nucleus

Fig. 4.7 The role of CD4 and CD8 in T-cell receptor (TCR)–major histocompatibility complex (MHC) antigen interaction. CD4 or CD8 is closely associated with the TCR complex. They bind MHC in a restricted fashion (CD8 to class I only, CD4 to class II only). Binding is antigen dependent and strengthens the bond between TCR and a complementary peptide-MHC complex. Molecules associated with CD4 or CD8 are then able to transduce a signal.

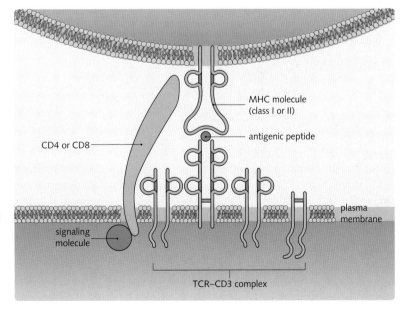

MHC molecule (class I or II)

antigenic peptide

CD4 or CD8

plasma membrane

signaling molecule

TCR–CD3 complex

21

Chromosomal location of BCR and TCR receptor segments and number of functional V, D, and J segments				
Gene	Chromosome	V	D	J
BCR heavy chain	14	51	27	6
BCR lambda light chain	22	40	0	6
BCR kappa light chain	2	40	0	5
TCR alpha	14	54	0	50
TCR beta	7	42	2	13
TCR delta	14	8	3	4
TCR gamma	7	6	0	5

Fig. 4.8 Chromosomal location of BCR and TCR receptor segments and number of functional V, D, and J segments (BCR, B-cell receptor; TCR, T-cell receptor; V, variable; D, diverse; J, joined).

Light-chain rearrangement then occurs in immature B cells. This process is illustrated in Fig. 4.10. Only after both rearrangements have occurred is an immunoglobulin BCR seen on the surface.

Allelic exclusion

This is the process whereby a B cell expresses only one set of heavy-chain genes and only one set of light-chain genes, thus ensuring that the antigenic specificity of the two halves of the Ig molecule is the same and that any B cell expresses immunoglobulin of only one specificity. Production of a functional heavy or light chain prevents rearrangement of the other sets of genes.

Junctional diversity

Several mechanisms are employed to create further diversity within the variable regions.

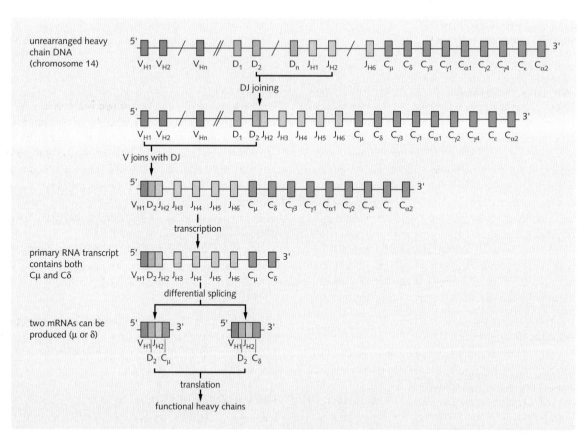

Fig. 4.9 Rearrangement of the heavy chain is similar to that of the light chain, although the join between D and J segments occurs first. In an unstimulated B cell, the heavy-chain mRNA that is transcribed contains both the Cμ and the Cδ segments. The mRNA can be differently spliced such that both IgM and IgD will be produced. They will both exhibit the same antigen-binding capacity.

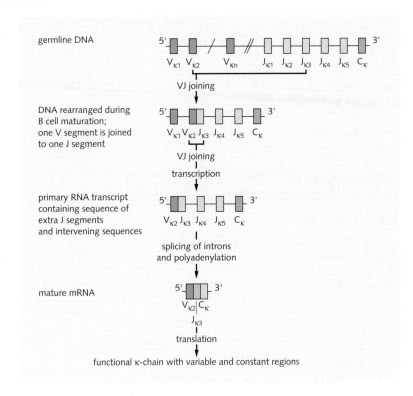

germline DNA

DNA rearranged during
B cell maturation;
one V segment is joined
to one J segment

VJ joining

transcription

primary RNA transcript
containing sequence of
extra J segments
and intervening sequences

splicing of introns
and polyadenylation

mature mRNA

translation

functional κ-chain with variable and constant regions

Fig. 4.10 Rearrangement of gene segments in the κ light chain. This process occurs during B-cell maturation and is not reversible.

Junctional flexibility and N-nucleotide addition

When exons are spliced, there are slight variations in the position of segmental joining. In addition, up to 15 nucleotides can be added to the D–J and the V–DJ joints. This occurs only in heavy chains and is catalyzed by terminal deoxynucleotidyl transferase.

Both junctional flexibility and N-nucleotide addition can disrupt the reading frame, leading to nonfunctional rearrangements. However, formation of productive rearrangements increases antibody diversity. The V–J, V–DJ, and VD–J joints fall within the antigen-binding region of the variable domain. Therefore, diversity generated at these joints will impact on the antigen specificity of the Ig molecule.

Somatic hypermutation

During the course of a primary immune response, point mutations occur in the variable region exons of the Ig molecule. The resultant Ig molecules may have altered affinity for antigen. Those with higher affinities are positively selected because of clonal antigen drive. Antibodies produced later in the primary immune response, and in the secondary immune response, will therefore have an increased affinity for antigen (affinity maturation).

Class switching

This is the process whereby a single B cell can produce different classes of Ig that have the same specificity. The mechanism is not well understood but involves "switch sites"—DNA sequences located upstream from each heavy-chain C-gene segment (except Cδ). Possible mechanisms include the following:

- Differential splicing of the primary transcript (see Fig. 4.9).
- A looping out and deletion of intervening heavy chain C gene segments (and introns).
- Exchange of C gene segments between chromosomes.

This process underlies the class switch from IgM in the primary response, to IgG, IgA, or IgE in the secondary response. Cytokines are important in controlling the switch.

TCR rearrangement

TCR chain recombination occurs in a manner analogous to BCR recombination in most T cells (the αβ cells). The β-gene rearrangement (D-J joining, then DJ-V joining) occurs first in the pre-T cell, followed by the α-chain rearrangement

(V–J joining) in the immature T cell. In the much less common γδ T cells, rearrangements of both genes appear to occur simultaneously.

The TCR does not exhibit somatic hypermutation. This is probably because T cells do not recognize self-peptides and only recognize self-MHC. Therefore, diversity is generated only in developing T cells, which can be deleted if they are either self-reactive or nonfunctional.

Humoral immunity

B cells and antibody production

The humoral immune response is brought about by antibodies, which are particularly efficient at eliminating extracellular pathogens. Antigen can be cleared from the host by a variety of effecter

mechanisms, which are dependent on antibody class or isotype:
- Activation of complement, leading to lysis or opsonization of the microorganism.
- Antibody-dependent cell-mediated cytotoxicity (ADCC).
- Neutralization of bacterial toxins and viruses.
- Mucosal immunity (IgA-mediated).

Activated and differentiated B cells, known as plasma cells, produce antibodies. An overview of B-cell activation is given in Fig. 4.11. B cells are activated within follicles found in secondary lymphoid structures (e.g., lymph nodes and spleen). B cells become activated only if they encounter specific antigen. During proliferation, variable regions of the immunoglobulin genes undergo somatic hypermutation. This process occurs in

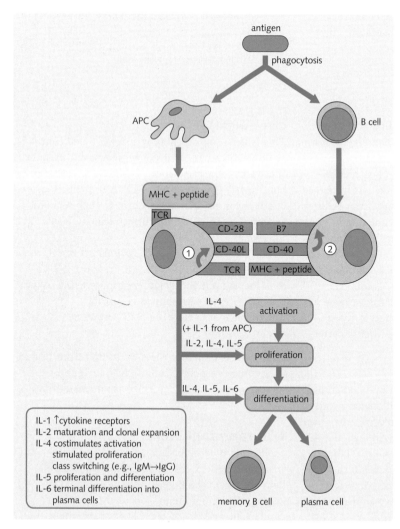

Fig. 4.11 Overview of the humoral immune response. Activated and differentiated B cells, known as plasma cells, produce antibody. B cells are activated by antigen in a T-cell-independent or T-cell-dependent fashion (only T-cell-dependent antigens are shown). T helper cells are primed by antigen-presenting cells (APCs), which present antigen in conjunction with MHC class II molecules. B cells are stimulated by antigen interacting with B-cell receptors. Primed T helper cells interact with B cells that also express antigen-MHC complexes. This interaction induces a sequence of surface receptor binding and cytokine production that results in B-cell activation, proliferation, and differentiation. (1) Binding of the T-cell receptor (TCR) to MHC induces the T cell to produce CD-40L, which binds to CD-40 on the B cell, producing a major stimulatory signal. (2) CD-28 on the T cell then interacts with B7 on the B cell (costimulatory signal). Cytokines are also involved; their actions are shown in the diagram.

the germinal center of the follicle. Follicular dendritic cells present antigen, to which the B-cell clones with the highest affinity will bind. This causes the expression of bc 1–2, which prevents B cells from undergoing apoptosis. Therefore, the highest-affinity clones are positively selected. B cells that respond to soluble antigen or do not receive T-cell help undergo apoptosis—negative selection of self-reactive and nonreactive clones. An overview of clonal selection of B cells is given in Fig. 4.12.

T-cell-dependent and T-cell-independent antigens

The process, shown in Fig. 4.11, illustrates the need for T cells in the activation of a humoral response. The antigens that trigger this process are therefore known as T-cell-dependent antigens. Not all antigens require T cells to produce an antibody response. T-cell-independent antigens, including many microbial constituents, are able to stimulate B cells directly or with the help of non–thymus-derived accessory cells.

Structure and function of antibody

The structure of immunoglobulin is shown in Fig. 4.13. Immunoglobulin molecules (using IgG as an example) are composed of two identical heavy and two identical light chains, linked by disulphide bridges. The light chains consist of one variable and three or four constant domains, depending on the class of antibody. Digestion of IgG with papain produces two types of fragment:

- Two Fab fragments (bind antigen) consisting of the light chain and two domains of the heavy chain (denoted VH and CH1).
- One Fc fragment (binds complement) consisting of the remainder of the heavy chain (CH2 and CH3).

The light chain
The light chain comprises two domains:
- The amino (N) terminal domain is variable and is the site of antigen binding.
- The constant domain at the carboxy (C) terminal.

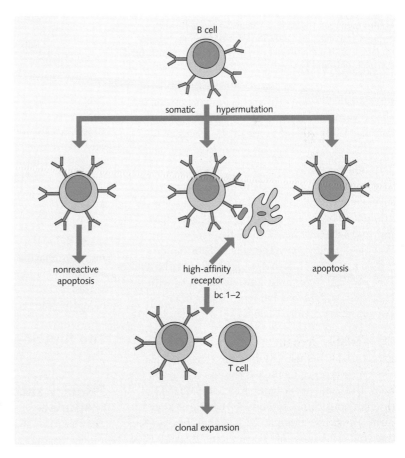

Fig. 4.12 Clonal selection of B cells. During B-cell activation, the antigen-binding region of the immunoglobulin gene undergoes hypermutation. Clonal selection ensures that cells that produce the best antibody are selected and that nonfunctional or self-reactive B cells are deleted. This process occurs within the germinal centers of lymphoid follicles.

25

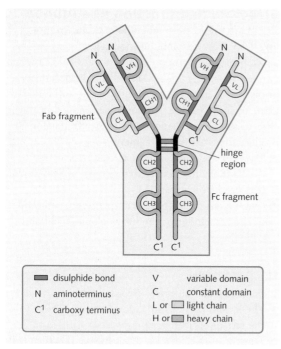

Fig. 4.13 Structure of IgG. Immunoglobulins are composed from two identical light and two identical heavy chains. The chains are divided into domains, each of which is an immunoglobulin fold. The variable domains form the antigen-binding site. Digestion of the immunoglobulin molecule with papain produces an Fc portion (which binds complement) and two Fab portions (which bind antigen).

The constant region can be κ or λ, but both light chains within an Ig molecule will be the same; approximately 60% of human light chains are κ.

The heavy chain

The heavy chain has a variable domain attached to several constant domains. There are five classes of immunoglobulin (Ig) in humans, IgG, IgA, IgM, IgE, and IgD. The heavy chain determines the immunoglobulin class. The heavy chain can be γ (IgG), α (IgA), μ (IgM), ε (IgE), or δ (IgD). IgG, IgA, and IgD have three constant domains with a hinge region; IgM and IgE have four constant domains but no hinge region.

The variable domain

Each variable domain exhibits three regions that are hypervariable. The hypervariable regions on both light and heavy chains are closely aligned in the immunoglobulin molecule. Together, they form the antigen-binding site and therefore determine the molecule's specificity. Because they must be complementary to the epitope they bind to, the hypervariable regions can be referred to as the complementarity-determining regions.

The hinge region

The hinge is a peptide sequence located between the first and second constant domains in the heavy chain. It allows the Fab regions to move against the Fc region from 0 to 90 degress. This allows greater interaction with epitopes. The hinge region is also the site of the interchain disulphide bonds.

Classes of antibody

Different classes and subclasses of antibody are known as **isotypes** or **allotypes**.
The **idiotype** of an antibody is the way the unique features of the variable domains function as epitopes (**idiotopes**), which will bind a variety of **anti-idiotype** antibodies.
Haptens are small molecules that need to be bound to a large carrier molecule to be immunogenic.

The different properties of the immunoglobulin classes are shown in Fig. 4.14. Different Ig classes and subclasses are specific to each species. IgG, IgE, and IgD are monomeric; secreted IgA (sIgA) is usually present as a dimer, and secreted IgM as a pentamer. The sIgA molecule is made up of two IgA monomers, a J chain and a secretory piece. The IgA dimer (+J chain) is produced by submucosal plasma cells and enters the mucosal epithelial cell via receptor-mediated endocytosis, binding to the poly-Ig receptor. Having passed from the basal to the luminal surface of the epithelial cell, the IgA dimer is secreted across the mucosa, with part of the poly-Ig receptor (the secretory piece) still attached.

The functions of antibodies

The functions of Igs are shown in Fig. 4.15.

Primary and secondary antibody responses

The first time that an antigen is encountered, there is a longer lag phase before antibody is produced, and

Properties of the five immunoglobulin classes					
	IgG	IgA	IgM	IgE	IgD
Physical properties					
Molecular weight (kDa)	150	300	900	190	150
Serum concentration (mg/mL)	13.5	3.5	1.5	0.0003	0.03
Number of subunits	1	2	5	1	1
Heavy chain	γ	α	μ	ϵ	δ
Subclasses	4	2	—	—	—
Biologic activities					
Present in secretions	✗	✓	✓	✗	✗
Crosses placenta	✓	✗	✗	✗	✗
Complement fixation	✓	✓	✓✓✓	✗	✗
Binds phagocytic receptors	✓	✗	✓	✗	✗
Binds mast cell receptors	✗	✗	✗	✓	✗
Other features					
Main role	Main circulatory Ig for secondary immune response	Major Ig in secretions	Main Ig in primary immune response	Allergy and antiparasitic response	Expressed on naïve B cell; function not known

Fig. 4.14 Properties of the five immunoglobulin (Ig) classes.

Functions of immunoglobulin	
Function	**Notes**
Opsonization	Phagocytic cells have antibody (Fc) receptors; thus, antibody can facilitate phagocytosis of antigen
Agglutination	Antigen and antibody (IgG or IgM) clump together because immunoglobulin can bind more than one epitope simultaneously. IgM is more efficient because it has a high valency (10 antigen-binding sites)
Neutralization	Binding to pathogens or their toxins prevents their attachment to cells
Antibody-dependent cell-mediated cytotoxicity (ADCC)	The antibody–antigen complex can bind to cytotoxic cells (e.g., cytotoxic T cells, NK cells) via the Fc component of the antibody, thus targeting the antigen for destruction
Complement activation	IgG and IgM can activate the classical pathway; IgA can activate the alternative pathway
Mast cell degranulation	Cross-linkage of IgE bound to mast cells and basophils results in degranulation
Protection of the neonate	Transplacental passage of IgG and the secretion of sIgA in breast milk protect the newborn

Fig. 4.15 Summary of the functions of immunoglobulins (sigA, secretory immunoglobulin A; NK, natural killer).

27

IgM is produced before IgG (primary response). The second and subsequent exposures result in a more rapid response of IgG only, which is of higher affinity and titer (secondary response). The primary and secondary responses are illustrated in Fig. 4.16.

Cell-mediated immunity

Cell-mediated immunity is mediated by T lymphocytes, macrophages, and natural killer (NK) cells. The cell-mediated immune system is involved in the elimination of the following:

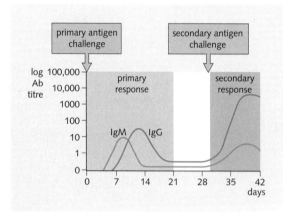

Fig. 4.16 Primary and secondary antibody (Ab) responses. IgM is the first antibody to be produced and is usually less specific than IgG that is produced subsequently. Following a second challenge with the same antigen, IgG is the primary antibody produced. It has a higher affinity for the antigen and is produced more rapidly in greater titers; in addition, high levels persist for longer than in the primary response. Less IgM is produced during the secondary response.

- Intracellular pathogens and infected cells.
- Tumor cells.
- Foreign grafts.

The thymus plays an important role in cell-mediated immunity because it is the site of T-cell maturation.

The thymus gland
The thymus is important for the production of T lymphocytes. T-lymphocyte differentiation begins in the bone marrow before early precursor cells migrate to the thymus. In the thymus, immature T lymphocytes undergo random recombination of their T-cell receptor genes. Some of the resulting T-cell receptors will be specific for pathogens and others for normal self-antigens. The role of the thymus is to select T cells that will respond to pathogens but not self-antigens.

The thymus is a gland with two lobes, located in the anterior part of the superior mediastinum—posterior to the sternum and anterior to the great vessels and upper part of the heart (Fig. 4.17). It can extend superiorly into the roof of the neck and inferiorly into the anterior mediastinum. It receives its blood supply from the inferior thyroid and internal thoracic arteries. Each lobe is surrounded by a capsule and divided into multiple lobules by fibrous septa known as trabeculae. Each lobule is divided into two regions (Fig. 4.18):
- An outer cortex.
- An inner medulla.

Immature thymocytes (T-cell progenitors) enter the thymus gland via the cortex, where they rapidly proliferate and rearrange their T-cell receptor genes. T cells that recognize self-antigen in the thymus are

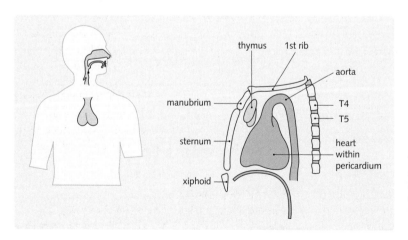

Fig. 4.17 Location of the thymus. The thymus is located in the superior mediastinum, behind the sternum but above and in front of the heart. It can extend into the neck. After puberty, the thymus reduces its size.

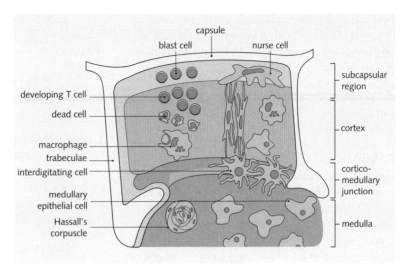

Fig. 4.18 Structure of a thymic lobule. The thymus is a bilobed gland, surrounded by a collagenous capsule, which is subdivided into lobules. Developing T cells (thymocytes) move from the subcapsular region to the medulla during maturation. Several different types of stromal cells support them. Many thymocytes undergo apoptosis (particularly in the cortex) and are phagocytosed by macrophages.

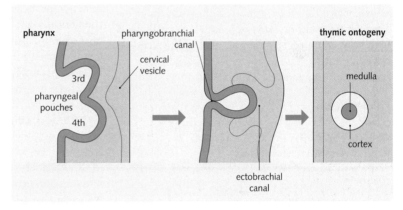

Fig. 4.19 Embryologic development of the thymus. The thymus develops from the third (and possibly fourth) pharyngeal pouch. This forms the medulla, which is surrounded by the ectobranchial canal formed from the cervical vesicle. The thymus is developed by 8 weeks of gestation.

forced to undergo apoptosis—negative selection. T cells that are able to bind MHC to some extent will proliferate—positive selection. A much smaller and more mature group of thymocytes survives to enter the medulla. Thymocytes continue to mature in the medulla and eventually leave the thymus, via postcapillary venules, as mature, antigen-specific, immunocompetent T cells. In total, only 1–5% of thymocytes in the thymus reach maturity; the remainder undergo programmed cell death (apoptosis).

Stromal cells of the thymus

The remainder of the thymic lobule is composed of a network of epithelial cells, known collectively as stromal cells. They interact with developing thymocytes and produce several hormones that are essential for their differentiation and maturation.

Embryologic origin of the thymus

The human embryonic thymus develops from the third pharyngeal pouch during week 4 or 5 of gestation (Fig. 4.19). The thymus gland is formed by week 8 and is fully differentiated and producing viable lymphocytes by week 17. The third pharyngeal pouch also gives rise to the parathyroid glands. Lymphoid stem cells are produced by the fetal liver and spleen, and by bone marrow from 6 months' gestation.

Thymic hypoplasia

Although it continues to grow until puberty, the relative size of the thymus gland decreases over this period. After puberty, there is a real reduction in size, and, by adulthood, it is composed largely of adipose tissue and continues to produce far fewer T lymphocytes.

T lymphocytes
Functions of different T-cell phenotypes
The different types of T cell can be differentiated by cell-surface molecules and function. There are two different types of T-cell receptor (TCR), which have different functions. T cells expressing αβ-TCRs account for at least 95% of circulatory T cells. They become cytotoxic, helper, or suppressor cells and, unless specified otherwise, account for all the T cells mentioned in this book. T cells expressing a γδ-TCR are present at mucosal surfaces, and their specificity is biased towards certain bacterial and viral antigens. Some γδ-T cells can recognize antigen independently of an APC. These T cells are usually cytotoxic in their actions. They differ from NK cells because they detect antigen rather than the presence or absence of MHC class I molecules. They are part of the adaptive system, because their action is specific and shows evidence of immunologic memory.

T helper cells
T helper (Th) cells play a key role in the development of the immune response:
- They determine the epitopes that are targeted by the immune system via their interactions with antigen in conjunction with class II MHC molecules on APCs.
- They determine the nature of the immune response directed against target antigens (e.g., cytotoxic T cell response or antibody response).
- They are required for normal B-cell function.

Most Th cells are CD4[+] and can be divided into four subsets on the basis of the cytokines they secrete:
1. Th0.
2. Th1.
3. Th2.
4. Treg.

Th0 cells arise as a result of initial short-term stimulation of naïve T cells; they are capable of secreting a broad spectrum of cytokines. Prolonged stimulation results in the emergence of Th1 and Th2 subsets. The cytokines released by the Th1 and Th2 subsets modulate one another's secretion. The different cytokine profiles of the Th1 and Th2 subsets reflect their different immunologic functions (Fig. 4.20). The fourth type of helper T cell has a regulatory role. If autoreactive T cells manage to escape negative selection in the thymus, they need to be inhibited in the peripheral tissues. Regulatory T cells are capable of preventing this immune response. Their action is unknown but is thought to be via cytokines, including transforming growth factor-β, IL-5, IL-6, and IL-10.

Cytotoxic T cells
Most cytotoxic T (Tc) lymphocytes are CD8[+] and recognize antigen in conjunction with class I MHC molecules (endogenous antigen). They lyse target cells via the same mechanisms as NK cells.

Development of T cells
T-cell precursors are produced in the bone marrow and are transported to the thymus for development

Differences between Th1 and Th2 cells		
	Th1 cells	Th2 cells
Cytokines secreted	IL-2, IL-3, IFN-γ, TNF-β	IL-3, IL-4, IL-5, IL-10, IL-13
Functions	• Responsible for classical cell-mediated immunity reactions such as delayed-type hypersensitivity and cytotoxic T cell activation	• Promote B-cell activation
	• Involved in responses to intracellular pathogens	• Involved in allergic diseases and responses to helminthic infections
	• Activate macrophages	• Induce rise in IgE and eosinophil levels

Fig. 4.20 Differences between the T helper 1 (Th1) and T helper 2 (Th2) cell subsets.

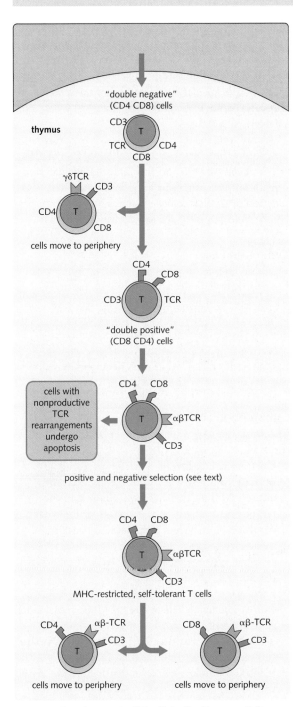

Fig. 4.21 Development of T cells in the thymus. Cells entering the thymus to become T cells are negative for CD4, CD8, CD3, and the T-cell receptor (TCR). Rearrangement of the genes encoding the TCR will produce three cell lines: (1) CD4$^+$ αβ- TCR; (2) CD8$^+$ αβ-TCR; and (3) CD4$^-$CD8$^-$ γδ TCR. The β or γ chain genes rearrange first. If a functional β chain is formed, both CD4 and CD8 are upregulated, and the α-chain gene rearranges. The resultant T cells are positively selected if

and maturation. The aim of T-cell development and maturation is to select T cells with receptors that can recognize foreign antigens in conjunction with self-MHC. Cells with nonfunctioning receptors or that are strongly self-reactive are destroyed (Fig. 4.21).

Positive selection

Positive selection occurs in the thymic cortex. T cells that are capable of binding self-MHC molecules are selected. These T cells also become MHC restricted. Developing T cells express both CD4 and CD8 until they become MHC restricted, when either CD4 or CD8 is downregulated. They interact with class I and class II MHC molecules, on thymic epithelial cells. T cells that do not interact with the MHC molecules undergo apoptosis, as they do not receive a protective signal as a result of the TCR–MHC interaction.

Negative selection

T cells that are positively selected but have high affinity for MHC molecules and self-antigen undergo negative selection. T cells with high affinity for self-MHC interact with MHC molecules on dendritic cells and macrophages, and are forced to undergo apoptosis.

T-cell activation

T cells are activated by interactions between the TCR and peptide bound to MHC. Activation also requires a "second message" from the antigen-presenting cell. This process is shown in Fig. 4.22. Once T cells are activated, they produce a wide range of molecules with several functions. These are primarily cytokines, which may be pro- or anti-inflammatory (see Fig. 4.20) or involved in activation of other immune cells.

Superantigens

T cells can be activated in a nonspecific fashion by superantigens. Superantigens cross-link between the V-β domain of the TCR and a class II MHC molecule on an antigen-presenting cell. Cross-linking is independent of the peptide binding cleft but depends on the framework region of the V-β domain. This means that one superantigen is able to activate

their TCR is functional but negatively selected if they react too strongly. The majority of the thymocytes will undergo apoptosis due to positive or negative selection (MHC, major histocompatibility complex).

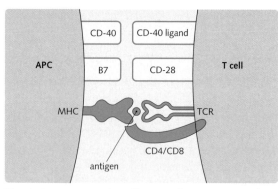

Fig. 4.22 Activation of T cells. Several interactions with antigen-presenting cells (APCs) are required to activate T cells. The T-cell receptor (TCR) and CD4 or CD8 bind to MHC and antigen. CD-28 on the T cell binds to B7 on the APC, providing a costimulatory signal (MHC, major histocompatibility complex).

about 5% of T cells, far more than normal antigen. An example of a T cell superantigen is staphylococcal enterotoxin.

Superantigens result in polyclonal activation, effectively "crowding-out" the specific, protective immune response. A consequence of polyclonal activation can be autoimmune disease. Superantigens can also result in the deletion of a large number of T cells by inducing negative selection in the thymus.

Secondary lymphoid organs

Lymphatic drainage and lymph nodes

Lymph nodes are secondary lymphoid organs. They provide a site for lymphocytes to interact with antigen and other cells of the immune system.

At the arterial end of capillaries, water and low-molecular-weight solutes leak out into tissue spaces to create interstitial fluid. Most interstitial fluid returns to the venous circulation at the venous end of capillaries (due to pressure gradients). The remainder leaves the interstitial space via the lymphatic system. Once interstitial fluid has entered a lymphatic vessel, it is known as lymph. Lymphatic vessels are present in almost all tissues and organs of the body.

Lymphatic circulation

The lymphatic system acts as a passive drainage system to return interstitial fluid to the systemic circulation; lymph is not pumped around the body. Lymph vessels, therefore, contain numerous valves to prevent backflow of lymph. Afferent lymph vessels carry lymph into lymph nodes. They empty into the subcapsular sinus, and lymph percolates through the node. Each node is drained by only one efferent vessel.

Lymph returns to the circulation at lymphovenous junctions. These are located at the junction of the right subclavian vein and right internal jugular vein (which empties the right lymphatic duct) and at the junction of the left subclavian vein and left internal jugular vein (which empties the thoracic duct).

Lymph nodes

Lymph nodes act as filters, "sampling" lymphatic fluid for bacteria, viruses, and foreign particles. Antigen-presenting cells (APCs), loaded with antigen, also migrate through lymph nodes. They are present throughout the lymphatic system, often occurring at junctions of the lymphatic vessels. Lymph nodes frequently form chains and may drain a specific organ or area of the body.

Lymph node structure

The structure of lymph nodes can be divided into three areas (Fig. 4.23):
- **Cortex:** mainly B cells, initially organized as primary follicles. B cells sample antigen from interstitial fluid that has been drained in the lymph and trapped on the surface of follicular dendritic cells. When stimulated by antigen, secondary follicles form, each containing a germinal center that produces large numbers of plasma cells and memory B cells.
- **Paracortex:** T cells and dendritic cells (APCs expressing high levels of class II MHC molecules). Activation of T cells (by antigen presented by dendritic cells and B cells) and interaction with B cells are needed to produce antibodies.
- **Central medulla:** cellular cords that are populated with B and T lymphocytes, plasma cells, and macrophages. The cords are located around medullary sinuses. The lymph drains into a terminal sinus, which eventually forms the efferent lymphatic vessel.

Lymph nodes act as sites for initiation of the adaptive immune response. Antigen is sampled, processed, and presented by several APCs (macrophages and dendritic cells).

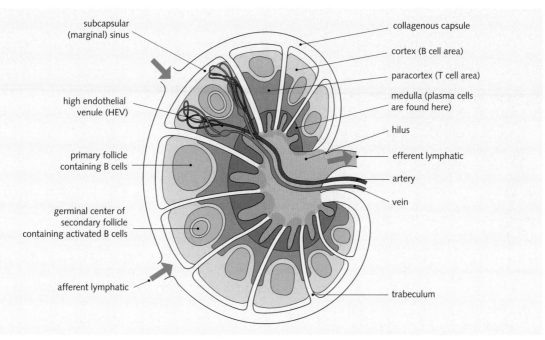

Fig. 4.23 Lymph node structure. A collagenous capsule through which several afferent lymphatic vessels pass surrounds lymph nodes. Lymph is deposited in the subcapsular sinuses and then drains through the cortex and paracortex and into the medulla, where it drains into the efferent lymph. The blood supply to the lymph node consists of an artery and a vein through which lymphoid cells can pass. The lymph node provides a good environment for initiation of an adaptive immune response.

Lymphocyte recirculation

Lymphocytes move continuously between blood and lymph. Efferent lymph contains more lymphocytes than afferent lymph because:

- Antigenic challenge results in stimulation and proliferation of lymphocytes.
- Lymphocytes enter the lymph node directly from blood.

Lymphocyte recirculation is essential for a normal immune response (Fig. 4.24). Approximately 1–2% of the lymphocytic pool recirculates each hour. This increases the chances of an antigenically committed lymphocyte encountering complementary antigen.

Lymphocytes tend to recirculate to similar tissues. For example, an activated lymphocyte that has migrated from the skin to a local lymph node is most likely to migrate to another lymph node draining skin following transport in the blood. Similarly, lymphocytes activated in mucosal-associated lymphoid tissue (MALT) will return to MALT. This recirculation is governed by the expression of molecules on both the lymphocyte and the surface endothelium. Areas of endothelium through which lymphocytes migrate are known as high endothelial venules (HEVs). Lymphocytes activated in MALT express α4β7 integrins that interact with MadCAM-1, an adhesion molecule only expressed on HEV in MALT tissue.

Mucosal-associated lymphoid tissue

MALT consists of unencapsulated subepithelial lymphoid tissue found in the gastrointestinal, respiratory, and urogenital tracts (Fig. 4.25). It can be subdivided into:

- Organized lymphoid tissue (e.g., tonsils, appendix, Peyer's patches).
- Diffuse lymphoid tissue located in the lamina propria of intestinal villi and lungs.

Organized lymphoid tissue
Respiratory tract

MALT tissue in the nose and bronchi includes the following:

- Lingual, palatine, and nasopharyngeal tonsils.
- Adenoids.
- Bronchial nodules.

33

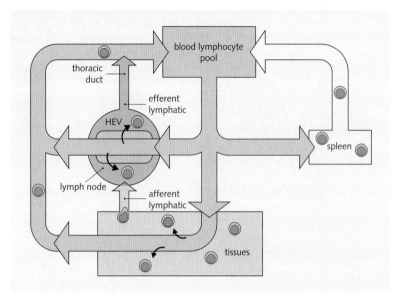

Fig. 4.24 Lymphocyte recirculation. Lymphocytes can enter lymph nodes via specialized high endothelial venules or in lymph. They leave the node in lymph that is returned to the systemic circulation via the right lymphatic duct or thoracic duct (HEV, high endothelial venule).

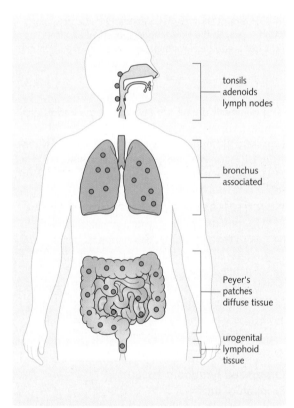

Fig. 4.25 Anatomic location of mucosal-associated lymphoid tissue (MALT). MALT is found in the nasal cavity, throat, respiratory tract, gastrointestinal tract, and urogenital tract. Immune cells activated in MALT will home only to other mucosal sites.

The respiratory system is exposed to a large number of organisms every day, most of which are cleared by the mucociliary escalator. Microorganisms that are not removed are presented by dendritic cells in the bronchi and stimulate germinating centers.

Gastrointestinal tract

Peyer's patches are organized submucosal lymphoid follicles present throughout the large and small intestine, being particularly prominent in the lower ileum. The structure of a Peyer's patch is shown in Fig. 4.26.

Lymphocyte trafficking in MALT

Mucosal lymphocytes generally recirculate within the mucosal lymphoid system. This occurs through recognition between specific adhesion molecules on the surfaces of lymphocytes from Peyer's patches and corresponding ligands on the venular endothelium.

The spleen

The spleen is a secondary lymphoid organ. It is the site of B- and T-cell proliferation and of antibody formation and an important component of the reticuloendothelial system. It is specialized to filter blood much as the lymph nodes filter lymph. Blood supply to the spleen is via the splenic artery. Blood is drained via the splenic veins, which join the superior mesenteric vein to form the portal vein.

The spleen is an intraperitoneal organ; its relations include the following:

- Anteriorly: the stomach, tail of the pancreas, and left colic flexure.
- Medially: the left kidney.
- Posteriorly: the diaphragm, left pleura, left lung, and ribs 9–11.

Structure

The spleen is surrounded by a dense, irregular fibroelastic connective tissue capsule that projects fibers known as trabeculae into the organ. The two main types of tissues found within the spleen are red pulp and white pulp. These are separated by a marginal zone (Fig. 4.27).

Red pulp

The red pulp is made up of venous sinuses and splenic cords. The splenic cords are composed of reticular fibers, reticular cells, plasma cells, phagocytes, and some B cells. The red pulp removes old or defective erythrocytes and platelets from the circulation.

White pulp and marginal zone

The central arteriole is surrounded by a periarteriolar lymphoid sheath (PALS), which

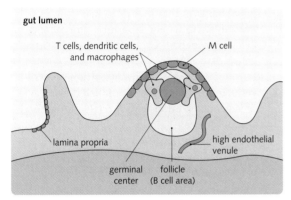

Fig. 4.26 Structure of a Peyer's patch. Peyer's patches are found in the gastrointestinal tract. Microbes are transported across specialized epithelial M cells in pinocytotic vesicles into a dome-shaped area. Antigen-presenting cells then process and present antigen to T cells. Helper T cells then activate B cells within the follicle.

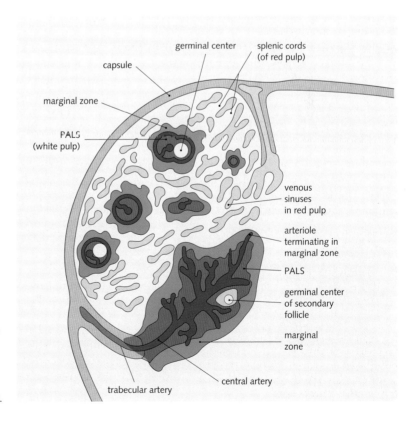

Fig. 4.27 Structure of the spleen. Arterioles entering the spleen are surrounded by T lymphocytes, the periarteriolar lymphoid sheath (PALS). Along with B cells organized into follicles, this constitutes the white pulp. These structures are surrounded by a marginal zone containing plasma cells, lymphocytes, macrophages, and dendritic cells. The rest of the spleen is composed of splenic cords (red pulp) and venous sinuses.

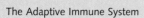
predominantly contains T cells. These branch between B-cell follicles that could be primary (unstimulated) but will be secondary (stimulated) in most patients. The PALS and follicles constitute the white pulp. The white pulp is surrounded by a marginal zone containing plasma cells, T and B lymphocytes, macrophages, and dendritic cells. The marginal zone is supplied by venous sinuses that have gaps as wide as 2–3 μm between the endothelial cells. The following functions occur in the marginal zone:

- Antigen-presenting cells sample blood for antigens.
- Lymphocytes exit the circulation and migrate to their respective domains.
- Monocytes enter the spleen and become macrophages. Here they can attack blood-borne microorganisms.
- Lymphocytes and dendritic cells come into contact, allowing initiation of an immune response.

The spleen also acts as a reservoir for platelets, erythrocytes, and granulocytes.

Embryology

The spleen begins as a mesodermal proliferation in the primitive gut during the fifth week of fetal development. It is connected to the body wall by the lienorenal ligament and to the stomach by the gastrolienal ligament.

Regulation of the Immune System

Several factors and interactions between the initiators and the mediators of the immune response determine the exact nature of the immune response and can augment it and limit it.

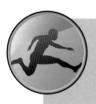

The nature of the immune response is regulated by antigen, interacting lymphocytes, and idiotype interactions.

1. Immune regulation by antigen and antigen presentation:
   - The nature of the antigen, the antigen dose, and the route of administration of the antigen are important in the determination of the response it elicits. Polysaccharide antigens are often T-cell independent and associated with mainly a humoral response, whereas protein antigens elicit both a humoral and a cellular response. Large antigen doses may cause tolerance. Subcutaneous and intradermal antigen administration favors a cellular response, whereas inhaled and intravenous administration favors a humoral response.
   - Antigen presentation is regulated by the level of MHC expression and the expression of adhesion and other accessory molecules.
2. Immune regulation by lymphocytes:
   - T-helper cell subsets regulate each other. Cytokines secreted by Th1 cells reduce Th2 cell activity, and cytokines secreted by Th2 cells reduce the activity of Th1 cells.
   - T-suppressor cells control B-cell activity. The mechanism is not fully elucidated; it may be that the T-suppressor cells are cytotoxic T cells reacting with the idiotype determinant of the antibody-producing cell.
3. Idiotype immune regulation:
   - Idiotypes (antigen structure of the variable region) can act as antigens if their immunoglobulin reaches a sufficient concentration. Anti-idiotype antibodies can react with the B cell producing the idiotype to cause cellular inactivation or complement-mediated lysis.
   - Anti-idiotype antibodies can also arise to the variable regions of the T-cell receptor and can cause T-cell control through binding, causing inactivation or complement-mediated lysis.

Neural and endocrine-mediated phenomena (e.g., corticosteroid secretion) can act to modulate the immune response.

- How is recognition molecule diversity generated?
- Why don't mature lymphocytes contain the full genome?
- Neither the T-cell receptor nor membrane immunoglobulin is able to signal. How do they transduce a signal?
- Why are there two classes of MHC? How do they relate to antigen presentation and cellular activation?
- What are the functions of different classes of immunoglobulins?
- How do lymphocytes recirculate? What is the relevance of this process?
- How does lymph node structure relate to function?
- What is mucosal-associated lymphoid tissue?
- What is the relevance of positive and negative selection of lymphocytes for the immune response?
- What are the differences between the different types of T helper cell?
- What are the factors that mediate the exact nature of an immune response?

FUNCTIONING OF THE IMMUNE SYSTEM

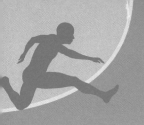

5. Inflammation and Healing of Damaged Tissues

Acute inflammation: stereotypical response of the innate immune system

Acute inflammation is the immediate response to cell injury. It is of short duration (a few hours to a few days) and is triggered by a range of insults, including chemical or thermal damage and infection. Infection is sensed by resident macrophages, which release chemokines and cytokines, attracting neutrophils to the site of infection. In other instances, inflammation is initiated by resident mast cells, which tend to attract eosinophils.

Once inflammation is initiated, several changes occur in vascular endothelium to allow attachment and extravasation of leukocytes—primarily neutrophils but also monocytes and lymphocytes. Attachment and extravasation require the presence of surface molecules on both the endothelium and leukocytes. The acute inflammation process is mediated by many different chemicals.

Vascular changes

Tissue injury results in the release of chemical mediators (cytokines, chemokines, and histamine) that act on local blood vessels. The main changes that occur include the following:

- Vasodilatation, which causes increased blood flow and, therefore, redness and heat.
- Slowing of the circulation and increased vascular permeability: formation of an inflammatory exudate results in swelling.
- Entry of inflammatory cells, especially neutrophils, into the tissues.

Leukocyte extravasation

Neutrophils adhere to the vessel wall and then pass between the endothelial cells into the tissues. This is a multistep process involving:

- Margination: adherence of neutrophils to the vessel wall (Fig. 5.1).
- Diapedesis (extravasation): neutrophils move between endothelial cells into the tissue.
- Chemotaxis: due to the release of several chemotactic agents (Fig. 5.2).

Integrin molecules allow immune cells to target specific sites (a process known as homing). To interact successfully with the extracellular matrix, neutrophils must express $\beta 1$-integrins, a set of adhesion molecules that can bind to collagen and laminin.

Fig. 5.1 Margination and extravasation (diapedesis) of neutrophils. Neutrophils adhere to vessel walls via cell adhesion molecules (CAMs). CAMs can be members of the immunoglobulin gene superfamily, the selection family, or the integrin family. Various inflammatory mediators modify the expression or alter the affinity of CAMs. Margination is a two-phase process that is followed by cellular migration (ICAM, intercellular adhesion molecule).

Margination and extravasation of neutrophils	
Margination	**Extravasation**
Phase I "Tethering and rolling" Weak interactions between: • L-selectin constitutively expressed on leukocytes • P- and E-selectin that are induced on endothelial cells	Further activator signals result in a conformational change in the leukocyte Metalloproteases are used to detach the cell from the endothelium, before if penetrates the endothelial basement membrane
Phase II "Activation and strengthening" • Rapid induction of integrins on leukocytes; (e.g., CD11b:CD18 [Mac-1] and CD11a:CD18 [LFA-1] on neutrophils) • Integrins bind to ICAM molecules expressed constitutively on endothelial cells Phase II is mediated by chemokines	

Mediators of acute inflammation	
Action	**Mediators**
Increased vascular permeability	Histamine, bradykinin, C3a, C5a, leukotrienes C_4, D_4, E_4, PAF
Vasodilation	Histamine, prostaglandins, PAF
Pain	Bradykinin, prostaglandins
Leukocyte adhesion	LTB_4, IL-1, TNF-α, C5a
Leukocyte chemotaxis	C5a, C3a, IL-8, PAF, LTB_4, fibrin and collagen fragments
Acute phase response	IL-1, TNF-α, IL-6
Tissue damage	Proteases and free radicals

Fig. 5.2 Overview of the mediators of acute inflammation (IL, interleukin; LT, leukotriene; PAF, platelet-activating factor; TNF, tumor necrosis factor).

Once neutrophils reach a site of inflammation, they phagocytose foreign particles and release enzymes. Leukocytes can release proteases and metabolites during chemotaxis and phagocytosis, which are potentially harmful to the host. Neutrophils die during this process, creating pus.

Chemical mediators of inflammation

Various chemical mediators are produced during an inflammatory response. They usually have short half-lives and are rapidly inactivated by a variety of systems. A summary of their actions is given in Fig. 5.2.

Histamine

Histamine is released from preformed granules within mast cells, basophils, and platelets. It increases vascular permeability and also causes vasodilatation.

Cell membrane phospholipid metabolites

Prostaglandins (PGs) and leukotrienes (LTs) are derived from the metabolism of arachidonic acid. Platelet-activating factor (PAF) is also an important mediator (Fig. 5.3).

Complement and kinins

The active fragments generated by the complement cascade, C3a and C5a, participate in increasing vascular permeability and chemotaxis. Proteolytic enzymes act acutely on plasma proteins to release peptide fragments called kinins. Bradykinin is the most notable kinin; it increases vascular permeability and mediates pain. The coagulation and fibrinolytic systems also play a minor role.

Cytokines

Cytokines IL-1, IL-8, and tumor necrosis factor alpha (TNF-α) are released from macrophages and effect local and systemic inflammatory responses.

Local effects include the following:
- Induces cell adhesion molecules (CAMs) on endothelium.
- Attracts neutrophils to area of injury.

Systemic effects include the following:
- Acts on hypothalamus to cause fever and anorexia.
- Affects marrow to mobilize neutrophils (elevates white cell count).
- Acts on liver to produce acute phase proteins (CRP, MBP, SAP).
- Acts on fat and muscle, effecting protein and energy metabolism.
- Activates the initial stages of the adaptive immune system.

Results of acute inflammation

The acute inflammatory response can quickly and effectively destroy the causative stimulus, after which changes resolve. If the stimulus cannot be cleared, chronic inflammation ensues. Leakage of enzymes and oxidative molecules can also damage tissue in the areas of acute inflammation and lead to the need to "heal" tissue damage.

Chronic inflammation

Chronic inflammation arises when the acute inflammatory stimulus cannot be cleared. It differs from the acute inflammation in several ways, as shown in Fig. 5.4.

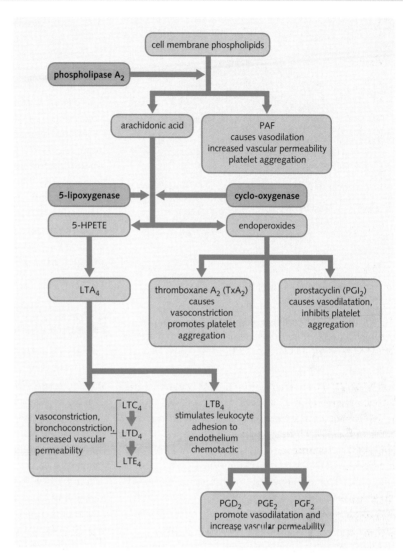

Fig. 5.3 Metabolism of membrane phospholipids in acute inflammation (LT, leukotriene, PAF, platelet-activating factor; PG, prostaglandin).

Acute versus chronic inflammation		
	Acute	Chronic
Cells involved	Neutrophils Monocytes	Altered macrophages Lymphocytes
Mediators	Kinins, complement, prostaglandins, and leukotrienes	T-cell and macrophage cytokines
Characteristic lesion	Abscess (liquifactive necrosis with neutrophils)	Granuloma (caseous necrosis with epitheliod cells and giant cells)

Fig. 5.4 Comparison of acute and chronic inflammation.

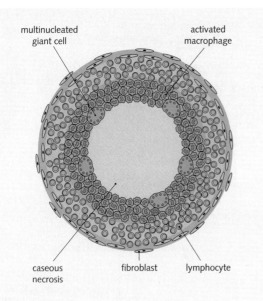

multinucleated giant cell

activated macrophage

caseous necrosis

fibroblast

lymphocyte

Fig 5.5 A granuloma, showing typical focal accumulation of lymphocytes and macrophages around a central area of caseous necrosis.

Antigenic persistence results in the continued activation and accumulation of macrophages. This leads to the formation of epithelioid cells (slightly modified macrophages) and granuloma formation (Fig. 5.5). TNF-α is needed for granuloma formation and maintenance. Interferon-γ (IFN-γ), released by activated T cells, causes macrophage transformation into epithelioid and multinucleate giant cells (which arise from the fusion of several macrophages). The granuloma is surrounded by a cuff of lymphocytes, and the migration of fibroblasts results in increased collagen synthesis. Caseous necrotic

areas (dry, "cheese-like" white mass of degenerated tissue) might be present in the center of a granuloma.

The nature of the damaging stimulus determines the type of granuloma formed. Inert particles (e.g., silica in the lungs) are predominantly surrounded by macrophages. Microorganisms such as *Mycobacterium tuberculosis* (which causes tuberculosis) induce a persistent, delayed-type hypersensitivity (DTH) response, resulting in granuloma formation in the lung and possibly leading to cavitation. The granuloma formed is characterized by focal accumulation of lymphocytes and macrophages. Phagocytosis is not usually effective because the microorganism can survive and multiply within macrophages. The granulomatous response, although preventing spread of infection, is harmful to the host.

Healing of damaged tissues

The nature of the healing process observed after an injury depends on the extent of the tissue damage and the type of the tissue involved by the injury. Tissues may be characterized as labile (constantly turning over), stable (proliferating when stimulated), and permanent (cells cannot renew themselves). If there has been no cell killing in the tissue, all tissues can return to their normal state by resolution of the inflammatory response. If cell killing has occurred, permanent tissues can heal only by repair via scarring. Labile and stable tissues can repair damage by regeneration if the damage has not been so severe that the underlying connective tissue has been destroyed. If the scaffolding is destroyed, these tissues too undergo repair by scarring. An overview of the process is summarized in Fig. 5.6.

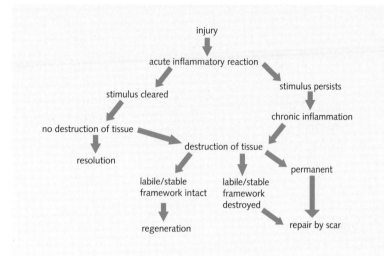

Fig. 5.6 From injury to healing.

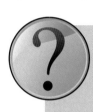

- What vascular changes are associated with acute inflammation?
- What process occurs for neutrophils to extravasate at sites of inflammation?
- Which chemicals mediate acute inflammation?
- What are the consequences of acute inflammation?
- What are the consequences of chronic inflammation?
- What are the components of the healing process?

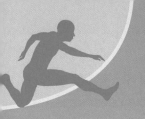

6. Immune Response to Pathogens

Viruses do not always kill host cells, but budding and release of new viral particles often cause the cells to lyse. The immune system can act to prevent infection or spread of infection or to eliminate an intracellular target once infection has occurred.

Humoral immunity to viruses

The humoral response is involved in preventing entry into, and viral replication within, cells.

Antibody

Antibodies can bind to free virus and prevent its attachment and entry into a cell (neutralization of virus particles). Antibodies can also bind to viral proteins expressed on the surface of infected cells. Antibody bound to cells can initiate antibody-dependent cell-mediated cytotoxicity (ADCC) and complement activation, and it acts as an opsonin for phagocytes.

Responses directed against free virus are considered to be the most important *in vivo*, and antibodies are therefore important early in the course of infection to prevent spread of virus between cells.

Interferon

Interferons (IFNs) are produced by virally infected cells. IFN-α and IFN-β act on neighboring uninfected cells and inhibit transcription and translation of viral proteins. IFN-γ activates macrophages and natural killer (NK) cells, and it enhances the adaptive immune response by upregulating expression of major histocompatibility complex (MHC) class I and class II molecules.

Cell-mediated immunity to viruses

Cell-mediated mechanisms are important for eliminating virus once infection is established. The cells involved include the following:

- NK cells: These are cytotoxic for virus-infected cells and participate in ADCC.
- Cytotoxic CD8$^+$ T cells: Viral peptides are presented on the cell surface in association with class I MHC molecules. CD8$^+$ T cells can destroy these infected cells.
- CD4$^+$ T cell: T helper cells are required for the generation of antibody and cytotoxic T cell responses, and the recruitment and activation of macrophages (Th1 help).

An overview of the immune response to viruses is given in Fig. 6.1.

Examples of viral infection and strategies to avoid immunity

Viral infections are common, and most are self-limiting. Some, particularly those that can evade the immune response, can be chronic and are potentially fatal (e.g., human immunodeficiency virus [HIV] and hepatitis B). Different viruses use different strategies to evade the host's immune response:

- Antigenic shift and drift: mechanisms of antigenic variation (e.g., influenza).
- Polymorphism (e.g., adenovirus, rhinovirus).
- Latent virus (e.g., herpes simplex virus [HSV], varicella-zoster).
- Modulation of MHC expression: cytomegalovirus (CMV), adenovirus, Epstein-Barr virus (EBV), herpes simplex virus (HSV), HIV.
- Infection of lymphocytes (e.g., HIV, measles, CMV).
- Prevention of complement activation (e.g., HSV).

Antigenic variation, either by mutation or polymorphism, circumvents immunologic memory because the virus expresses different immunologic targets. By becoming latent, virus "hides" from the immune system. Latent virus often reactivates when the immune system is compromised, suggesting that there must be some interaction between the immune system and the virus, even when it is latent. Mechanisms that prevent normal effector functions from being carried out primarily involve downregulation of MHC class I expression. However, viruses can also interfere with IFN or produce inhibitory cytokines. Infection of

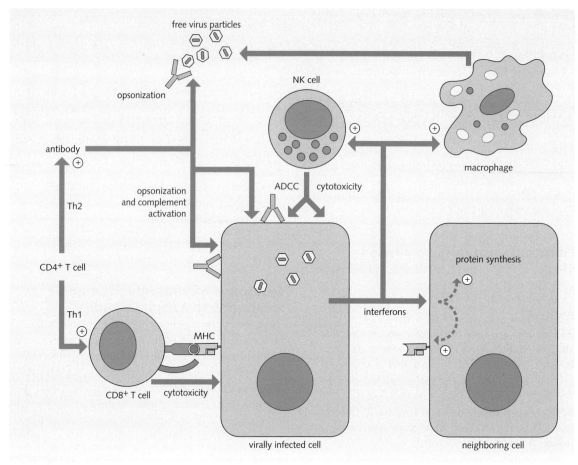

Fig. 6.1 The immune response to virus. Interferons, produced by virally infected cells, have three important actions. Interferon-α and interferon-β induce an antiviral state in neighboring cells (inhibition of viral transcription and translation). Interferon-γ activates macrophages and natural killer (NK) cells and upregulates major histocompatibility complex (MHC) molecules. NK cells kill virally infected cells either by detecting the absence of MHC class I molecules or by antibody-dependent cell-mediated cytotoxicity (ADCC). Macrophages phagocytose opsonized free virus and cell fragments and produce further interferon. CD8$^+$ (cytotoxic) T cells sense viral peptides presented by MHC class I molecules and destroy the cell. CD4$^+$ (helper) T cells help to activate macrophages and are involved in the generation of antibody and cytotoxic T-cell responses.

lymphocytes and their death reduce the ability of the immune system to combat viral infection.

Immune response to bacterial infection

Bacteria are prokaryotic organisms. Their cell membrane is surrounded by a peptidoglycan cell wall. Many bacteria also have a capsule of large, branched polysaccharides. Bacteria attach to cells via surface pili, but only some bacteria enter host cells. Different immune mechanisms operate, depending on whether the bacteria are extracellular or intracellular.

Extracellular bacteria
Humoral immunity to extracellular bacteria
Complement
Bacteria activate complement via the lectin or alternative pathways. Activated complement products play a role in the elimination of bacteria, especially C3b (an opsonin), C3a, and C5a (anaphylatoxins that recruit leukocytes) and the membrane attack complex (MAC), which can

perforate the outer lipid bilayer of gram-negative bacteria.

Lysozyme

Lysozyme is a naturally occurring antibacterial that attacks N-acetyl–muramic acid–N-acetyl glucosamine links in the bacterial cell wall. This results in bacterial lysis.

Antibody

This is the principal defense against extracellular bacteria:

- sIgA binds to bacteria and prevents their binding to epithelial cells.
- Antibody neutralizes bacterial toxins.
- Antibody activates complement.
- Antibody acts as an opsonin.

Cell-mediated immunity to extracellular bacteria

Phagocytic cells kill most bacteria; C3b and antibody enhance phagocytosis. Bacterial antigens are processed and presented, in conjunction with class II MHC molecules, on the surface of APCs, to CD4$^+$ T cells. CD4$^+$ T cell help is required for the generation of the antibody response (Th2 help).

An overview of the immune response to extracellular bacteria is given in Fig. 6.2.

Intracellular bacteria
Humoral immunity to intracellular bacteria

The humoral mechanisms that are employed against extracellular bacteria will be used to try to prevent bacteria from causing intracellular infection. However, they will not be effective once the infection is intracellular.

Cell-mediated immunity to intracellular bacteria

Cell-mediated immunity is very important in the defense against intracellular bacterial infections, such as those caused by *M. tuberculosis*:

- Macrophages attempt to phagocytose the bacteria. If the organisms persist, chronic inflammation will ensue. This can lead to delayed (type IV) hypersensitivity.
- Cells infected with bacteria can activate NK cells, which cause cytotoxicity and can activate macrophages.
- CD4$^+$ T cells release cytokines that activate macrophages (Th1 help).

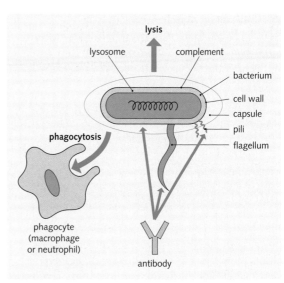

Fig. 6.2 The immune response to extracellular bacteria. The first line of host defense against bacteria is lysozyme. This "natural antibiotic" attacks N-acetyl–muramic acid–N-acetyl glucosamine links in the bacterial cell wall. This, together with complement, leads to bacterial lysis. Antibody is produced against flagella (thus immobilizing bacteria) and pili (thus preventing attachment). Capsular polysaccharides can induce T-cell-independent antibody. Antibodies aid complement activation and phagocytosis of bacteria.

- CD8$^+$ T cells recognize antigens presented in conjunction with class I MHC molecules on the surface of infected cells and lyse these cells.

Examples of infection and bacterial strategies to avoid immunity

Bacterial strategies to avoid the immune response must include one of the following:

- Prevent phagocytosis.
- Allow survival within phagocytes.
- Prevent complement activation.
- Avoid recognition by the immune system.

Strategies to avoid immunity include the following:

- Inhibition of phagocytosis by capsules (e.g., *Streptococcus pneumoniae*, *Haemophilus* spp.).
- Killing of phagocytes by toxins (e.g., *Staphylococcus* spp.).
- Neutralization of opsonizing IgG (e.g., *Staphylococcus* spp.).
- Survival within phagocytes (e.g., *M. tuberculosis*, *Mycobacterium leprae*, *Toxoplasma* spp.).

49

- Inhibition of complement activation (e.g., *Staphylococcus* spp., *Streptococcus* spp., *Haemophilus* spp., *Pseudomonas* spp.).
- Polymorphism (e.g., *Streptococcus pneumoniae*, *Salmonella typhi*).

Like viruses, bacteria can be highly polymorphic. Bacteria of the same species can appear to be entirely different to the immune system.

Immune response to protozoal infection

Protozoa are microscopic, single-celled organisms. Fewer than 20 types of protozoa infect humans, although malaria, trypanosomes, and *Leishmania* cause significant morbidity and mortality. Protozoa cause intracellular infection, have marked antigenic variation, and are often immunosuppressive. They have complex life cycles, with several different stages, and therefore present the immune system with a variety of challenges. Protozoal infection is often chronic, since the immune system is not very efficient at dealing with these organisms. Most of the pathology of protozoal disease is caused by the immune response.

Humoral immunity against protozoa

Complement and antibody are important during the extracellular stage of infection. This opsonizes the protozoa and can cause lysis or prevent infection.

Cell-mediated immunity against protozoa

- **Phagocytosis** by macrophages, monocytes, and neutrophils is an important part of the immune response against protozoa.
- **CD4$^+$ T cells** are activated in response to protozoal infection. The subset of CD4$^+$ T cells activated is thought to determine whether the immune response is protective or not. T helper 1 cytokines (e.g., IL-2, IFN-γ, TNF-β) are considered protective.
- **Cytotoxic CD8$^+$ T cells** are important in destroying protozoa that replicate within cells (e.g., the sporozoite stage of *Plasmodium falciparum*, which causes malaria).
- **NK cells and mast cells** are often activated in protozoal infection.

Examples of protozoal infection and evasion of the immune response

Protozoa have good mechanisms to prevent the initiation of an immune response. Strategies include the following:

- Escape into the cytoplasm following phagocytosis (e.g., *Trypanosoma cruzi*).
- Prevention of complement actions (e.g., *Leishmania* spp.).
- Gene switching to create antigen variation (e.g., trypanosomes).
- Immunosuppression (e.g., trypanosomes).

- Outline the immune response to viral infection.
- Outline the immune response to extracellular and intracellular bacterial infection.
- Outline the immune response to protozoal infection.
- Identify the mechanisms that pathogens use to evade the immune response.

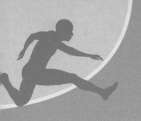

7. Hypersensitivity Mechanisms

Concepts of hypersensitivity

Hypersensitivity is an exaggerated or inappropriate immune response that causes tissue damage (immunopathology). The antigens involved are often innocuous. The mechanisms used to eliminate antigen under normal circumstances can cause damage to normal tissues (hypersensitivity). Hypersensitivity can take place in response to the following:

- An infection that cannot be cleared (e.g., tuberculosis).
- A normally harmless exogenous substance (e.g., pollen).
- An autoantigen (e.g., DNA in systemic lupus erythematosus [SLE]).

Hypersensitivity reactions have been classified, by Gell and Coombs, into four types: I, II, III, and IV. Types I, II, and III are antibody mediated; type IV is cell mediated.

Type I hypersensitivity

In type I (or immediate) hypersensitivity, the antigen (allergen) induces a humoral IgE immune response. On first exposure to the allergen, an individual produces specific IgE. IgE binds to high-affinity Fc-ε receptors (receptors for the Fc portion of the IgE molecule) on mast cells and basophils. Upon subsequent exposures, cross-linking of membrane-bound IgE induces release of mast cell granules. Their effects can be localized or systemic (Fig. 7.1).

Mast cell granule contents		
Mediator		**Action**
Primary	Histamine	Increased capillary permeability, vasodilation, smooth muscle contraction
	Serotonin	Increased capillary permeability, vasodilation, smooth muscle contraction, platelet aggregation
	Heparin	Anticoagulation, modulates tryptase
	Proteases — Tryptase	Activates complement (C3)
	Proteases — Chymase	Increased mucus secretion
	Eosinophil chemotactic factor	Chemotactic (cells move towards site of production) for eosinophils
	Neutrophil chemotactic factor	Chemotactic for neutrophils
	Acid hydrolases	Degradation of extracellular matrix
	Platelet-activating factor	Platelet aggregation and activation, increased capillary permeability, vasodilation, chemotactic for leukocytes, neutrophil activation
Secondary	Leukotrienes (C_4, D_4, B_4)	Vasodilation, smooth muscle contraction, mucus secretion, chemotactic for neutrophils
	Prostaglandins (D_2)	Vasodilation, smooth muscle contraction, chemotactic for neutrophils, potentiation of other mediators
	Bradykinin	Increased capillary permeability, vasodilation, smooth muscle contraction, stimulation of pain nerve endings
	Cytokines	Various

Fig. 7.1 Mast cell mediators and their actions. Mast cells contain many preformed (primary) mediators that are stored in granules. They can also synthesize new (secondary) mediators when they are activated.

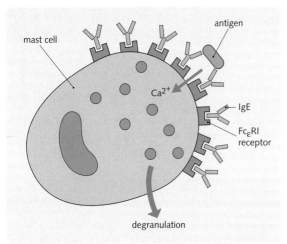

Fig. 7.2 Activation of mast cells by immunoglobulin E (IgE). IgE, produced by plasma cells, binds via its Fc domain to receptors on the mast cell surface. Cross-linking of these receptors by an antigen causes an influx of calcium ions into the cell. Calcium ions cause a rapid degranulation of inflammatory mediators from the mast cell.

The immune mechanisms of type I reactions are illustrated in Fig. 7.2.

Examples of type I reactions include the following:

- Allergic rhinitis (hay fever): pollens.
- Allergic asthma: house-dust mite.
- Systemic anaphylaxis: penicillin, peanuts, or insect venom.

> Atopy is a genetic predisposition to produce IgE in response to many common, naturally occurring allergens. It has a prevalence of 10–30%. Atopic patients can suffer from multiple allergies. The genetic basis of atopy is not known.

Type II hypersensitivity

Type II (or cytotoxic) hypersensitivity occurs when antibody specific for cell surface antigens is produced. Cell destruction can then result via:

- Complement activation.
- Antibody-dependent cell-mediated cytotoxicity (ADCC).
- Phagocytosis.

The immune mechanisms of type II hypersensitivity reactions are summarized in Fig. 7.3.

Examples of type II reactions in which complement is activated and cells destroyed are:

- Incompatible blood transfusions.
- Hemolytic disease of the newborn.
- Autoimmune hemolytic anemias.

Several diseases are caused by antibody directed against cell surface receptors, which can stimulate or block the receptor. In Graves' disease, stimulating antibodies are directed against the receptor for thyroid-stimulating hormone. In myasthenia gravis, blocking antibodies are directed against the acetylcholine receptor.

Type III hypersensitivity

In type III (or immune-complex-mediated) hypersensitivity, antibody combines with soluble antigen. The resulting immune complexes are usually phagocytosed but, if they persist, can cause immune complex disease (Fig. 7.4).

The immune complexes can be deposited in tissues near the site of antigen entry (localized type III reaction). This is demonstrated by the Arthus reaction, in which an intradermal or subcutaneous injection of antigen into a recipient with high levels of appropriate circulating antibody produces localized immune complexes that activate complement and generate acute inflammation.

Localized type III reactions are exemplified by:

- Farmer's lung: repeated inhalation of actinomycetes found in moldy hay.
- Pigeon-fancier's disease: repeated inhalation of antigens found in dried pigeon feces.

If immune complexes form in blood, they circulate around the body and are deposited in the blood vessel walls of a number of tissues, especially the kidneys and joints (generalized type III reaction). Systemic type III reactions can cause autoimmune diseases such as SLE and occur in infectious diseases such as malaria and viral hepatitis.

Type IV hypersensitivity

Upon first contact with antigen, a subset of CD4$^+$ T-helper (Th) cells is activated and clonally expanded (this process takes 1–2 weeks). Upon subsequent encounter with the same antigen, sensitized Th cells

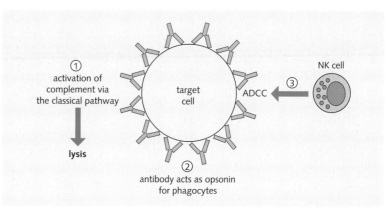

Fig. 7.3 The immune mechanisms of type II hypersensitivity reactions. Antibody bound to cells (either antibody to foreign cells or autoantibody) results in cell death via (1) complement, (2) phagocytes, or (3) natural killer (NK) cells (ADCC, antibody-dependent cell-mediated cytotoxicity).

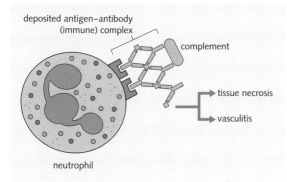

Fig. 7.4 The immune mechanisms of type III hypersensitivity reactions. Immune complexes that are normally removed by phagocytes are deposited in blood vessels or in tissues, resulting in severe damage via complement and neutrophils.

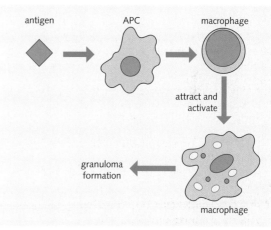

Fig. 7.5 The immune mechanisms of type IV hypersensitivity reactions. These reactions take several days to be initiated because antigen is first presented to T cells, which can then activate macrophages (APC, antigen-presenting cells).

secrete cytokines. These attract and activate macrophages, which account for more than 95% of the cells involved. Activated macrophages have increased phagocytic ability and can destroy pathogens more effectively. The type IV reaction peaks at 48–72 hours after contact with the antigen (time taken for the recruitment and activation of the macrophages) and is therefore known as delayed-type hypersensitivity. An overview of the immune mechanisms involved is given in Fig. 7.5.

Type IV reactions are important for the clearance of intracellular pathogens. However, if antigen persists, the response can be detrimental to the individual, as the lytic products of the activated macrophages can damage healthy tissues. Examples of antigens that induce a type IV response include the following:
- Contact antigens such as nickel and poison ivy.
- Intracellular pathogens such as *M. tuberculosis* and *Leishmania major*.

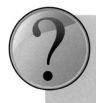

- Define hypersensitivity.
- Identify the immune mechanisms that result in hypersensitivity.
- Explain type I hypersensitivity.
- Explain type II hypersensitivity.
- Explain type III hypersensitivity.
- Explain type IV hypersensitivity.

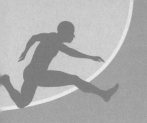

8. Clinical Evaluation of the Immune System

Clinicians are interested in detecting the presence of the immune response. A number of laboratory tests are used to assess the immune system.

Enumeration of immune system cells

The total and differential white blood cell count is a useful measure of immune activity. A change in the number of identifiable white cells in the blood can suggest an infectious or hypersensitivity state. Diseases associated with increases in white cell counts are illustrated in Fig. 8.1.

Decreases in the various types of white cells can indicate problems with immune function. Since all lymphocytes resemble each other morphologically, flow cytometry is often used to identify the numbers of specific types of lymphocytes.

Flow cytometry is a useful tool for differentiating between different populations of cells as well as for counting the number of cells within a sample. This is done by producing a very fine stream of medium, where only one cell at a time passes through a beam of laser light. Sensors detect when a cell blocks the beam of light, and the amount of light scatter identifies the size and granularity of the cell. Various surface antigens on the cell can be bound by monoclonal antibodies (specific for one antigen). The monoclonal antibodies are labeled with dyes that fluoresce under laser light (immunofluorescence). Different types of dye allow the detection of specific antigens (most machines use red and green fluorescence, but up to five colors are used by some machines).

CD antigens that are often used to characterize lymphocyte populations include the following:
- B cells: CD-19, CD-20, or CD-22.
- Helper T cells: CD2 or CD3 and CD4.
- Suppressor/cytotoxic T cells: CD2 or CD3 and CD8.
- Natural killer cells: CD2 and CD-16.

Other CD antigens can be assessed by flow cytometry to arrive at a cause for immune system failure. These include defects in adhesion molecules (CD-11/CD-18) and failures of B-cell class-switching (CD-40L).

Measurement of molecules associated with immune reactions

It is often useful to measure both total immunoglobulin levels and levels of specific types of immunoglobulins. Assays of total IgG, IgA, or IgM are based on specific immunopreciptin reactions either in gel diffusion or in fluid phase by nephelometry. Antibodies raised in animals against human immunoglobulins form complexes with immunoglobulins in the patient's serum. The distance of the precipitate that forms in the gel containing the anti-immunoglobulins from the well containing the serum or the amount of light scattered due to the formation of complexes detected in the liquid phase where anti-immunoglobulins are mixed with serum is proportional to the level of the particular immunoglobulin in the serum.

Total immunoglobulin levels vary with age. In a newborn, only maternal IgG transferred across the placenta is present; thus, immunoglobulin levels decrease and are at a nadir at 4 to 6 months of age. As the individual encounters more pathogens, levels of immunoglobulins increase with age, reaching adult levels at puberty. Approximate reference levels of total IgG, IgA, and IgM in the plasma are shown in Fig. 8.2.

Total IgE and amount of a specific type of antibody are present in concentrations that require the use of amplifying sandwich techniques. In all assays, the antigen of interest (anti-IgE or another specific antigen) is bound to a surface. The antigen is first incubated with serum; if antibody to the antigen is present, it will bind to the antigen. The surface is then washed, and antibody to human immunoglobulin conjugated with a detecting molecule is added (detecting substances include radioactive substances, enzymes, and fluorescent and luminescent molecules). If antibody from the serum has bound, the anti-immunoglobulin will bind to it.

The surface is then washed again, and reagents are added to quantify the amount of detecting molecules

Diseases associated with increases in white-cell count		
Cell type	**Associated diseases**	**Examples**
Leukocytes	Pathologic stress, leukemia	
Neutrophils	Bacterial infections	Pyogenic bacteria
	Acute inflammation or tissue necrosis	Infarction, surgery, burns, myositis, vasculitis
	Neoplasms	Carcinoma, lymphoma, melanoma
	Myeloproliferative disorders	Chronic myeloid leukemia, myelofibrosis
	Metabolic disorders	Eclampsia, gout, diabetic ketoacidosis
Eosinophils	Parasitic infestation	Malaria, hookworm, filariasis, schistosomiasis
	Allergic reaction	Asthma, hay fever
	Skin disease	Pemphigus, eczema, psoriasis, dermatitis herpetiformis, urticaria
	Neoplasms	Hodgkin's disease, metabolic carcinoma, chronic myeloid leukemia
	Infections	Convalescent phase of any infection
Basophils	Myeloproliferative disorders	Chronic myeloid leukemia, polycythemia rubra vera
Lymphocytes	Acute infections	Mononucleosis, pertussis, rubella, viral infection
	Chronic infections	TB, syphilis
	Neoplasms	Chronic lymphocytic leukemia, lymphoma
Monocytes	Chronic infections and inflammatory diseases	TB, bacterial endocarditis, protozoa
	Neoplasms	Lymphomas, myelodysplastic syndromes

Fig. 8.1 Diseases associated with increased white-cell counts (TB, tuberculosis).

(e.g., by counting radioactive decay, measuring the product of the enzyme reaction, or detecting fluorescence or luminescence).

Fig. 8.3 shows how an enzyme-linked immunosorbent assay (ELISA) functions. Evaluations of specific levels of IgE in relation to allergy-associated antigens and of IgG or IgM in relation to specific pathogens or antigens in a vaccine are quite useful in management of allergic and infectious diseases.

Functional tests of immunity

Antigens causing type I hypersensitivity can be assessed by skin-prick testing. A number of allergens (antigens) are injected into the skin. The development of a wheal-and-flare reaction in minutes indicates the presence of specific IgE directed against that antigen. There is a slight risk that, if IgE levels are very high, a life-threatening systemic reaction can occur.

Type IV hypersensitivity can also be studied by injecting purified antigen beneath the skin. If a cell-mediated response is present, the result is a raised red area (activated lymphocytes are aggregating and releasing cytokines) after 24–48 hours. The purified protein derivative (PPD) test for tuberculosis is an example of this type of testing.

White cells isolated from blood can be placed in *in vitro* test systems to assess their function.

Total Immunoglobulin levels (in mg/dL)			
Age	IgG	IgA	IgM
Newborn	800–1200	0–5	5–15
6 Months	200–600	10–50	25–65
3 Years	550–950	25–75	30–80
10 Years	900–1100	100–210	40–90
Adult	900–1500	150–275	75–125

Fig. 8.2 Total immunoglobulin levels (mg/dL) according to age.

Neutrophils can be activated and then their ability to reduce nitroblue tetrazolium (NBT) assessed. If the neutrophils are capable of generating radicals important in oxidative killing, clear NBT will be reduced to a blue color detectable under the microscope.

Lymphocytes can be isolated and incubated with general activators (lectins such as PHA or pokeweed mitogen) or specific antigens to see if they respond. Response is judged by the incorporation of radioactive DNA precursors, morphologic changes in the cell (blastogenesis), or the release by the lymphocytes into the culture media of cytokines, which are produced when lymphocytes are activated.

Direct immunofluorescence

A biopsy of tissue can be studied to determine whether antibodies are bound to tissue components (type II hypersensitivity) or immune complexes are deposited in the tissue (type III hypersensitivity).

Frozen sections are made of the tissue and then incubated with antihuman immunoglobulin and anticomplement antibodies, which are conjugated with fluorescent compounds. The tissue is washed to remove unbound fluorescent conjugated antibodies. It is then observed under a microscope with illumination that excites the fluorescent molecule for the deposition of the conjugated molecules.

Type II processes are usually associated with a uniform distribution of fluorescence, reflecting antibody adherent to the structure in question (e.g., basement membrane).

Type III processes are usually associated with granular deposits, reflecting the presence of discrete immune complexes.

Direct immunofluorescence is useful in the diagnosis of autoimmune diseases, as discussed later.

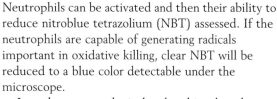

enzyme

monoclonal anti-IgG

specific IgG in patient's serum

viral antigen

plate

Fig. 8.3 Enzyme-linked immunosorbent assay (ELISA). ELISA can be used to detect antigens but is most commonly used to measure antibody to a specific antigen (e.g., a virus), as shown. Viral antigen is bound to plate, and the patient's serum is added. If specific IgG is present, it will bind to the antigen. Enzyme-labeled anti-IgG is added (binding to the patient's IgG). The enzyme converts a colorless substrate into a colored product. The intensity of color is relative to the amount of antigen.

- Explain the significance of a change in the number of white blood cells.
- Describe flow cytometry. Explain when it is used.
- Describe the amplifying sandwich techniques for measurement of immunoglobulin.
- Explain how ELISA can be used to diagnose the presence of an antigen in serum.
- Explain when skin-prick testing is used.
- Discuss the role of direct immunofluorescence in the detection of type II and type III hypersensitivity reactions.

9. Immune Deficiency

Immune deficiency predisposes individuals to infections from opportunistic pathogens (those that do not normally cause disease) as well as normal pathogens. Although the cause of the deficiency can be primary or secondary, the part of the immune system that is deficient will determine the sort of infection to which the individual is predisposed. Antibody deficits result in extracellular bacterial infection. T-cell deficiencies can result in viral, fungal, and intracellular bacterial infections.

Suspecting an immune deficiency

Knowing when to evaluate an individual for an immune deficiency requires careful assessment of clinical history. Evaluation for an immune deficiency should be considered in the following circumstances:
- Two or more episodes of pneumonia within 1 year.
- Recurrent deep skin or organ abscesses.
- Persistent yeast (*Candida*) infection beyond infancy.
- Two or more episodes of severe infections such as meningitis, osteomyelitis, or sepsis.
- Deep-seated infection with a classic opportunistic pathogen (e.g., *Pneumocystis carinii*).
- Failure to thrive in an infant or child.
- Need to use intensive (intravenous) antibiotics to clear a common infection (e.g., sinusitis).
- A family history of primary immunodeficiency.

Primary immune deficiencies

Primary immune deficiencies result from a genetically determined abnormality of immune function. The frequency of the different types of immune deficiency is as follows:
- Antibody deficiency: 50%.
- Cellular or combined cellular/antibody deficiency: 30%.
- Phagocyte (neutrophil) deficiencies: 18%.
- Complement deficiencies: 2%.

Antibody deficiencies

Major antibody deficiencies syndromes are:
- X-linked agammaglobulinemia (Bruton syndrome): due to a defect in Bruton tyrosine kinase. B cells and immunoglobulins are virtually absent. Affected boys present in infancy with recurrent pyogenic infections. Treatment is with intravenous immunoglobulin preparations.
- M-heavy chain deficiency: autosomal recessive condition due to a defect at the M-heavy chain locus (14q 32.2); clinically identical to Bruton syndrome.
- Selective IgA deficiency: this common condition (1 in 700 whites) may be asymptomatic or may be associated with recurrent respiratory or GI infections. It is due to a defect at the A-heavy chain locus on 14q and is a potential cause of anaphylaxis in patients transfused with plasma.
- X-linked hyper-IgM syndrome: demonstrates high levels of IgM but not other immunoglobulins. It is due to a defect in T cells. Because the CD-40 ligand is absent, immunoglobulin class-switching does not occur. Patients have recurrent pyogenic infections.
- Common variable hypogammaglobulinemia: onset later in life, which is associated with depression of immunoglobulin levels. The cause is unknown, but it is thought to result from a defect in T cell and/or B-cell regulation. It is treated with intravenous immunoglobulins.

Cellular and combined cellular/immunoglobulin deficiencies

Major cellular and combined cellular/immunoglobulin deficiencies are:
- Severe combine immunodeficiency (SCID): this is actually a number of conditions in which both B-cell and T-cell numbers are markedly reduced and immunoglobulins are not produced. Defects in any of several genes can lead to SCID. The most frequent cause is a mutation on the X chromosome that causes a deficiency of the common γ chain of cytokine receptors. Autosomal recessive forms of SCID result from mutations in receptor signaling pathways (e.g., Jak3 gene on

19p) or mutations in genes involved in nucleic acid metabolism (e.g., adenosine deaminase [ADA] or purine nucleoside phosphorylase [PNP] deficiency), which result in accumulation of toxic metabolites and inhibition of DNA synthesis.

- CD3 receptor defects: mutations in the genes that constitute the CD3 receptor result in a variable degree of immune deficiency manifest as a susceptibility to opportunistic infection. T-cell numbers are markedly decreased, whereas B cells and NK cells are detectable. Immunoglobulin levels are decreased.
- MHC receptor deficiency: mutations resulting in a failure of MHC I or MHC II molecules to combine with antigen result in a failure of presentation of antigens so that the adaptive immune system cannot respond. MHC II defects are more common than MHC I. Often, normal numbers of B, T, and NK cells are present, but MHC I or MHC II class molecules are not detected on cell surfaces by flow cytometry. Lymphocytes will respond to nonspecific mitogens but not to previously encountered antigens.

Some cellular immune deficiencies have distinctive combinations of clinical features:

- **DiGeorge syndrome** results from an error in embryogenesis of the third and fourth pharyngeal arches, causing failure of formation of the thymus and parathyroid glands and abnormalities of the cardiac great vessels. B and NK cells are present, but T cells are markedly decreased. Patients often present with hypocalcemia.
- **Wiskott-Aldrich syndrome** presents with eczema, thrombocytopenia, and decrease in T and B cells with age. Absent or decreased expression of WASP protein coded for on the X-chromosome is associated with cytoskeletal defects. Patients have an increased risk of opportunistic infections and immune cell neoplasms.

Phagocyte (neutrophil) defects

The most common neutrophil defect is neutropenia, which is usually not genetic but acquired. A condition called cyclic neutropenia causes individuals to experience episodes of neutropenia with a regular periodicity. There is increased risk of infection during periods of low counts. It is related to a defect in the elastase gene. Congenital conditions that lead to abnormal bone marrow development (reticular

dysgenesis) affect all immune cells, but neutropenia is often the first defect noted.

Functional abnormalities of neutrophils include:

- Leukocyte adhesion defect: this is due to an absence of CD11/CD18 (integrans) on the neutrophil membrane and results in a failure of adherence and diapedesis of neutrophils from vessels, causing a failure of acute inflammation.
- Chronic granulomatous disease: defects in the components of NADPH oxidase impair killing of ingested pathogens. The condition is most commonly X-linked but can be autosomal recessive. NBT tests are abnormal.

Complement defects

These are uncommon. All are associated with an abnormal result when one measures the ability of serum to lyse immunoglobulin-coated red cells (functional total hemolytic complement). Common complement deficiencies are listed in Fig. 9.1.

Management of primary immunodeficiency

The approach to management of primary immunodeficiency varies with the nature of the defect. Complement deficiency is usually managed with increased vigilance for the development of infection, as there is no practical source of complement other than plasma. Neutrophil defects are also managed by aggressive therapy when infection occurs. Some neutropenias (e.g., cyclic neutropenia) can be ameliorated by the use of

Primary complement deficiencies	
Disorder	**Features**
Deficiency of classical pathway components	Tend to develop immune complex disease
C3 deficiency	Prone to recurrent pyogenic infections
Deficiency of C5, C6, C7, C8, factor D, properdin	Increased susceptibility to *Neisseria* infections
C1 inhibitor deficiency	Causes hereditary angioedema

Fig. 9.1 Primary complement deficiencies. Deficiencies of almost all complement components have been described.

growth factor (G-CSF) therapy. T-cell and combined immunodeficiencies usually require a bone marrow stem cell transplant to restore normal immune function. An exception to this is DiGeorge syndrome, which can be managed with appropriately matched and processed thymic epithelial transplanted beneath the skin. B-cell immunodeficiencies are managed by supplying immunoglobulin. Two types of immunoglobulin preparations are available: a type that is administered intramuscularly and a form that can be given intravenously. Both are derived by fractionating plasma; the intravenous form then requires an additional step to chemically modify the immunoglobulin constant chain so that in the concentrated form immunoglobulins do not form aggregates that could cause serious reactions when infused. The characteristics of the two immunoglobulin preparations are summarized in Fig. 9.2.

> Cellular defects are managed by stem-cell transplant. Humoral defects are managed by infusion of immunoglobulins.

Both intramuscular immunoglobulin (ISG) and intravenous immunoglobulin (IVIG) are nearly completely IgG, so they are of no use in IgA deficiency. Since they are plasma derived, they at least theoretically could transmit a blood-borne

agent, although this has never been demonstrated to be an actual problem.

Secondary immune deficiencies

Malnutrition and disease
Lack of dietary protein and certain elements (e.g., zinc) predisposes to secondary immunodeficiency. Infections such as malaria and measles also result in immunodeficiency.

Malignancy
Secondary immunodeficiency is particularly common with tumors that arise from the immune system, such as myeloma, lymphoma, and leukemia. Many other tumors are immunosuppressive. This is likely to provide the tumor cells with a selective advantage, because they evade destruction by cytotoxic cells.

Steroids, other drugs, and radiation
Iatrogenic causes of immunosuppression are common. Immunosuppressive drugs can be given to suppress inflammatory or autoimmune disease or to prevent rejection of transplanted tissues. Radiation and cytotoxic drugs can be used to treat malignancies and frequently cause immunosuppression.

Acquired immunodeficiency syndrome (AIDS)
Human immunodeficiency virus (HIV), a retrovirus, is the causative organism of AIDS. In 2002, the worldwide prevalence of HIV infection was over

Fig. 9.2 Characteristics of the two immunoglobulin preparations.

Characteristics of the two immunoglobulin preparations		
Characteristic	ISG	IVIG
Use	High titer preparations for specific infections	Managed immune deficiency syndromes
Titers provided	Unreliable	Very high and predictable levels can be attained
Administration	Limited by discomfort of IM injection, given quickly in many settings	Closely monitored Infused slowly
Reaction risk	1/100 injections	1/20 infusions
Cost	Moderate	Expensive

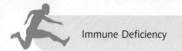

50 million people, and 5 million people died from AIDS. There are two types:

- HIV-1 has a worldwide distribution. The structure of HIV-1 is shown in Fig. 9.3.
- HIV-2 is confined mainly to West Africa. HIV-2 has lower transmission rate than HIV-1 and runs a more benign clinical course.

Both viruses mutate rapidly, so that an infected person can contain several different strains. Transmission of the virus takes place via three routes:

- Mucosal (i.e., by sexual contact): associated with other sexually transmitted diseases.

- Vertical: from mother to child (during the birth process and in breast milk, rarely transplacentally).
- Exposure to infected blood: intravenous drug abusers, blood transfusions, needlestick injuries (0.3% risk from single exposure).

The primary infection is often asymptomatic but can be marked by a flu-like illness (fever, macular rash, mouth ulcers, splenomegaly, and diarrhea) in 15% of individuals. This is followed by an asymptomatic period (median: 8–10 years). It was previously thought that HIV became latent during this period. However, it is now established that HIV replication rates during this phase of the infection are very high in the lymph nodes, resulting in the production of billions of viral particles per day. The immune system is capable of containing the infection during this phase, and the viral load (amount of HIV RNA in blood) in plasma remains low. Toward the end of the asymptomatic phase, individuals often develop persistent generalized lymphadenopathy. The final phase of the disease is AIDS, which is characterized by the following:

- A low CD4 count (less than 200 cells/µl).
- Opportunistic infections such as pneumonia due to *Pneumocystis carinii*, Cryptococcus, and cytomegalovirus infection.
- Neoplasia, in particular Kaposi's sarcoma (caused by herpesvirus 8) and B-cell lymphoma.
- Neurologic manifestations (due to the virus itself and as a result of opportunistic infection such as cerebral toxoplasmosis).

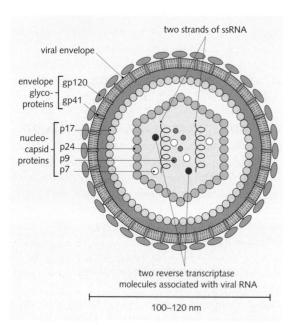

Fig. 9.3 Structure of HIV-1. The envelope glycoproteins gp120 and gp41 are hypervariable. gp120 binds CD4, allowing entry of the virus into the cell. The viral envelope is a lipid bilayer containing both viral glycoprotein antigens and host proteins.

Viral load and CD4 count vary throughout HIV infection, as illustrated in Fig. 9.4. The clinical features of AIDS relate to the CD4 count (Fig. 9.5).

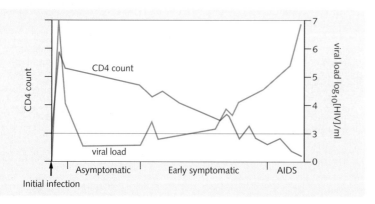

Fig. 9.4 Variation in CD4 count and viral load during the course of HIV infection.

Clinical infections at different CD4 counts	
CD4 count	Infection
<400	Tuberculosis
<300	Kaposi's sarcoma Esophageal candidiasis
<200	*Pneumocystis carinii* pneumonia (PCP) Toxoplasmosis
<100	*Mycobacterium avium intracellulare* CMV retinitis

Fig. 9.5 Clinical infections at different CD4 counts (CMV, cytomegalovirus).

Immunology of HIV infection

The gp120 antigen of HIV–1 binds the CD4 molecule on T helper (Th) cells, cells of the monocyte/macrophage lineage, and dendritic cells; gp41 is then required to enter the cell. Accessory receptors on immune cells, particularly the chemokine receptors CCR5 and CCR4, are also important. Infected monocytes, macrophages, and follicular dendritic cells in lymph nodes are thought to be the major reservoir for HIV. The following changes occur:

- Peripheral blood CD4$^+$ T cells are depleted.
- Defects in T-cell function are seen on both *in vivo* (failure to respond to recall antigens) and *in vitro* testing.
- Polyclonal B-cell activation occurs, resulting in hypergammaglobulinemia.
- Neutralizing antibodies directed against the gp120 and gp41 antigens are generated but do not prevent disease progression because of the high mutation rate of the virus.
- Cytotoxic T cells can prevent infection (rarely) or slow progression.

Detection of HIV infection

Screening for HIV infection is performed, using ELISAs to detect anti-HIV antibodies.

If the ELISA is positive, confirmatory tests must be carried out (e.g., a Western blot, which detects antibodies against specific HIV proteins). Seroconversion (production of antibodies) might not take place until 3 months after infection; hence, there is a window period when ELISA will be negative. This is a potential problem in blood transfusion.

In infants, anti-HIV IgG can be maternally derived and persist for up to 18 months, making diagnosis of HIV by ELISA unreliable. Detection of HIV by polymerase chain reaction (PCR) is used to confirm HIV infection in neonates.

Treatment of HIV

The treatment of HIV is now very successful. Although the infection cannot be cured, survival and quality of life have been profoundly increased. Treatment is with antiretrovirals and antibiotics:

- **Antiretroviral therapy:** antiretrovirals target HIV at various points of its life cycle (Fig. 9.6). HIV mutates rapidly and can become resistant to drugs. This is less likely to happen when combinations of different classes of antiretrovirals, known as highly active antiretroviral therapy (HAART), are used. HAART is usually initiated when viral load rises late in infection. It usually results in a reduction of viral load to undetectable levels and an increase in CD4 counts, with concomitant restoration of immune competence.
- **Antibiotic prophylaxis and treatment of infection:** prophylaxis against infections such as *Pneumocystis carinii* and *Toxoplasma gondii* is effective and usually given when the CD4 count is less than 200/µl. It has been shown that antibiotic prophylaxis can be safely stopped following immune restoration using treatment with HAART.

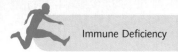
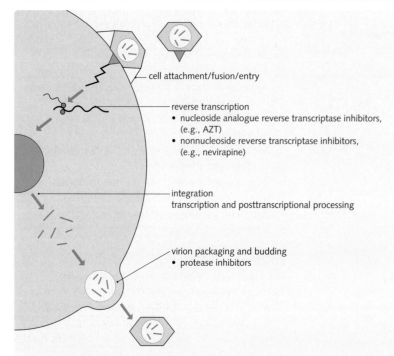

cell attachment/fusion/entry

reverse transcription
- nucleoside analogue reverse transcriptase inhibitors, (e.g., AZT)
- nonnucleoside reverse transcriptase inhibitors, (e.g., nevirapine)

integration
transcription and posttranscriptional processing

virion packaging and budding
- protease inhibitors

Fig. 9.6 Antiretroviral agents in current use and their site of action in the life cycle of HIV (AZT, azidothymidine).

- What are the causes and features of primary immunodeficiencies?
- What are the causes of secondary immunodeficiencies?
- What is the immunology of HIV infection?
- What are the laboratory features of HIV infection?
- How is HIV infection diagnosed?
- How is HIV infection treated?

10. Immunization

It is important to be able to explain the difference between active and passive immunity. Active immunity is produced by the body in response to antigen (either infection or vaccination). In vaccination, active immunity produces a response to antigen that is given to the patient. Preformed antibodies are used in passive immunization.

Immunity can be achieved by passive or active immunization (Fig. 10.1).

Active immunization

Active immunization results from contact with antigens, either through natural infection or by vaccination. Individuals exhibit a primary immune response, with clonal expansion of B and T cells and formation of memory cells. Subsequent exposure to the same antigen will induce a secondary immune response.

Vaccination

Vaccination is a form of active immunization that induces specific immunity to a particular pathogen. The aim is to produce a rapid, protective immune response on re-exposure to that pathogen. An ideal vaccine is:

- Safe, with minimal side effects and free from contaminating substances.
- Immunogenic, activating the required branches of the immune system, inducing long-lasting local and systemic immunity.
- Heat stable, because there are difficulties with refrigeration, particularly in tropical countries.
- Inexpensive, an important consideration, especially in developing countries.

Types of vaccine

The types of vaccine in current use are listed in Fig. 10.2. Most vaccines are live attenuated or killed; the features of each are compared in Fig. 10.3. The routine immunization schedule used in the United States is shown in Fig. 10.4. The most current schedule is available at www.cdc.gov/nip/.

Vaccines are not 100% efficacious. A small proportion of individuals receiving vaccination will not respond adequately. However, by immunizing the majority of the population, nonresponders are unlikely to come into contact with the virus because the viral reservoir is reduced (herd immunity).

It is possible to enhance the immune response to vaccines by using adjuvants. Adjuvants (e.g., aluminum salts and *Bordetella pertussis*) are nonspecific.

Comparison of passive and active immunity		
	Passive	**Active**
Features	Preformed immunoglobulins transferred to individual	Contact with antigen induces adaptive immune response
	Large amounts of antibody available immediately	Takes some time to develop immunity
	Short life span of antibodies	Long-lived immunity induced
Examples	Antitetanus toxin antibody	Natural exposure; vaccination

Fig. 10.1 Comparison of active and passive immunity.

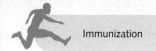
Different types of vaccine		
Vaccine	**Features**	**Examples**
Live attenuated	Attenuation achieved by repeated culture on artificial media or by serial passage in animals; immunogenicity is retained, but virulence is significantly diminished	Oral polio (Sabin), BCG, rubella, measles, mumps
Killed	Intact organisms killed by exposure to heat or chemicals (e.g., formalin)	Intramuscular polio (Salk), pertussis
Subunit	Purified, protective immunity-inducing antigenic components; often surface antigens	Influenza, pneumococcal
Recombinant	Genes encoding epitopes, which elicit protective immunity, are inserted into prokaryotic or eukaryotic cells; large quantities of vaccine are produced rapidly	Hepatitis B surface antigen (produced in yeast cells)
Toxoids	Bacterial toxins inactivated by heat or chemicals	Diphtheria, tetanus
Conjugates	Polysaccharide antigen is linked to protein carrier to enhance immunogenicity	*Haemophilus influenzae* type B (Hib), meningococcal

Fig. 10.2 Different types of vaccine in current use (BCG, bacille Calmette-Guérin).

Features of live versus killed vaccines		
Feature	**Live attenuated vaccine**	**Killed vaccine**
Level of immunity induced	High: organism replicates (mimicking natural infection)	Low: nonreplicating organisms produce a short-lived stimulus
Cell-mediated response	Good: antigens are processed and presented with MHC molecules	Poor
Local immunity	Good	Poor
Cost	Expensive to produce and administer	Cheaper than live vaccines
Reversion to virulence	Possible but rare	No (therefore safe for immunocompromised and pregnant patients)
Stability	Heat labile	Heat stable
Risk of contamination	Possible (e.g., by virus in cell media)	–

Fig. 10.3 Features of live vs. killed vaccines. The genes of attenuated organisms can differ from the wild type by just a few base pairs. It is relatively easy for them to mutate back to the disease-causing strain (MHC, major histocompatibility complex).

Contraindications to active immunization

While every effort is made to make sure that vaccinations are not only effective but very safe, there are certain contraindications to use of vaccines. The most important reasons not to immunize an individual include the following:

- Live attenuated vaccines should not be given to immunocompromised individuals.
- Individuals who experience severe allergic reactions to components of vaccines (e.g., egg protein, antibiotics) should not receive that vaccine.
- Individuals who have recently received immunoglobulin should not receive live attenuated vaccines (renders them potentially ineffective).
- In individuals with moderate or severe illness, with or without fever, immunizations should be

deferred until the individual is recovering and no longer acutely ill.

• Pregnant women should not receive live attenuated vaccines.

United States immunization schedule (standard-risk Individuals)	
Age	**Vaccine**
Birth	Hepatitis B
2, 4, and 6 months	DTaP, IPV, Hib, and PCV (hepatitis B at 2 months only)
12 to 15 months	Hepatitis B, DTaP, MMR, Hib, Varicella, PCV (influenza for 6 to 23 month olds)
4 to 6 years	DTaP, IPV, MMR
11 to 12 years	Td
College	Td, Mening (consider hepatitis A)
Adult	Influenza (>50 years old, yearly), PPV (>65 years old), Td (every 10 years), immunizations required for travel

Fig. 10.4 United States immunization schedule (DTaP, diphtheria and tetanus toxoid and acellular pertussis; IPV, inactivated polio virus (Salk); Hib, *Hemophilus influenzae* type B conjugate vaccine; PCV, pneumococcal conjugate vaccine; MMR, measles, mumps, and rubella vaccine; Td, tetanus and diphtheria toxoid; Mening, meningococcal polysaccharide vaccine; PPV, pneumococcal polysaccharide vaccine).

Passive immunization

Passive immunization involves the transfer of preformed immunoglobulins to an individual. Passive immunization is used if an individual requires rapid protection from an organism, venom, or toxin to which the individual is not immune. A number of passive immunization preparations are available (Fig. 10.5).

Immunization with DNA

A potentially valuable approach to immunization is the development of DNA vaccines. The process utilizes the DNA that encodes the antigen to which immunity is desired. This DNA is attached to a suitable promoter in a bacterial plasmid. The hypothesized mechanism for obtaining immunity is summarized in Fig. 10.6.

The advantages to this approach include low cost, vaccine stability, absence of a potentially infectious agent, and an immune response that mimics a natural infection. The one major disadvantage is the potential for integration of the DNA in the vaccine into the DNA of the host. Such disruption of an important host function may result in oncogenesis.

Passive immunization preparations	
Type of product	**Indications**
Immune globulin (derived from pooled human plasma)	Hepatitis A and measles prevention
Hyperimmune globulin (derived from selected high-titer human plasma)	Hepatitis B, rabies, tetanus, varicella, vaccinia, cytomegalovirus management
Specific monoclonal immune globulin	Respiratory syncytial virus (RSV) prevention
Equine immune globulin	Management of tetanus, botulism, spider and snake bites

Fig. 10.5 Passive immunization preparations. Use of the equine globulins involves significant risk of allergic reactions, and patients are often prick-tested or premedicated with steroids.

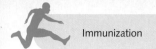

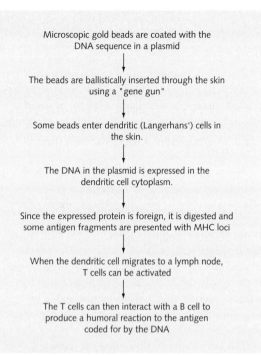

Microscopic gold beads are coated with the DNA sequence in a plasmid

↓

The beads are ballistically inserted through the skin using a "gene gun"

↓

Some beads enter dendritic (Langerhans') cells in the skin.

↓

The DNA in the plasmid is expressed in the dendritic cell cytoplasm.

↓

Since the expressed protein is foreign, it is digested and some antigen fragments are presented with MHC loci

↓

When the dendritic cell migrates to a lymph node, T cells can be activated

↓

The T cells can then interact with a B cell to produce a humoral reaction to the antigen coded for by the DNA

Fig. 10.6 Hypothesized mechanism for DNA immunization.

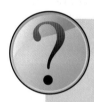

- List the differences between active and passive immunity.
- List the qualities of an ideal vaccine.
- Summarize the routine immunization schedule in the United States.
- Compare and contrast live and killed vaccines.
- Identify the contraindications to active immunization.

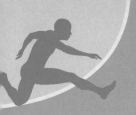

11. Allergy

Allergy is due to hypersensitivity reactions to exogenous antigens (known as allergens), mediated by IgE. Allergic symptoms usually result from degranulation of mast cells. This process is mediated by the cross-linking of IgE by allergen. Allergic conditions, therefore, are type I hypersensitivity reactions. Other types of hypersensitivity cause chronic forms of allergy. The symptoms of different allergies affect different tissues and can be local or generalized. Fig. 11.1 shows the spectrum of allergic conditions.

Asthma

Asthma is a chronic inflammatory disorder of the airways, characterized by reversible airflow obstruction. The airways become hyperresponsive, and exaggerated bronchoconstriction follows a wide variety of stimuli (e.g., exercise or cold air). The symptoms of asthma are cough, wheeze, chest tightness, and shortness of breath. Asthma is a common disease and is diagnosed in 5–10% of children. The incidence has risen over the past few decades, particularly in more economically developed countries.

Pollens, house-dust-mite feces, and animal fur are the most common allergens. These cause inflammation of the bronchial wall involving:
- Infiltration by eosinophils, mast cells, lymphocytes, and neutrophils.
- Edema of the submucosa.
- Smooth muscle hypertrophy and hyperplasia.
- Thickening of the basement membrane.
- Mucous plugging.
- Epithelial desquamation.

Asthma is diagnosed by a reversal in airway obstruction (measured by forced expiratory volume in the first second) of more than or equal to 15% following the administration of an inhaled β_2-adrenoreceptor agonist (such as salbutamol). This

Allergic reactions		
Allergic condition	**Common allergens**	**Features**
Systemic anaphylaxis	Drugs Serum Venoms Peanuts	Edema with increased vascular permeability Leads to tracheal occlusion, circulatory collapse, and possibly death
Acute urticaria	Insect bites	Local wheal and flare (red and raised)
Allergic rhinitis	Pollen (hay fever) Dust-mite feces (perennial rhinitis)	Edema and irritation of nasal mucosa
Asthma	Pollen Dust-mite feces	Bronchial constriction, increased mucus production, airway inflammation
Food	Shellfish Milk Eggs Fish Wheat	Itching urticaria and potentially anaphylaxis
Atopic eczema	Pollen Dust-mite feces Some foods	Itchy inflammation of the dermis and epidermis Usually red and sometimes vesicular

Fig. 11.1 Summary of allergic reactions.

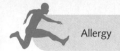

treatment is used for the short-term improvement of symptoms, although inhaled steroids and other immunosuppressive/anti-inflammatory drugs are used prophylactically to prevent asthma attacks.

Atopic/allergic eczema

Eczema or dermatitis can be caused by an allergic response. Dermatitis means skin inflammation. There are several types of dermatitis, including allergic eczema and contact dermatitis (a type IV hypersensitivity reaction). The reaction occurs wherever the allergen contacts the skin, but it can persist indefinitely. Contact dermatitis can be diagnosed by patch testing, and treatment is primarily by avoidance of the allergen.

Atopic eczema is most commonly the result of exposure to pollen or house-dust-mite feces. Common allergens are shown in Fig. 11.1. About 10% of children are diagnosed with eczema. Eczema commonly affects the flexural creases and the fronts of the wrist and ankles. In infancy and adulthood, the face and trunk are often involved. The skin lesions are itchy, red, and sometimes vesicular; they may be dry. Because of itching, the skin is often excoriated, which can lead to lichenification (thickening of the skin). Eczema is often complicated by superinfection with bacteria, particularly *Staphylococcus aureus*.

The diagnosis of atopic eczema is usually clinical. Total serum IgE, RAST for specific IgE, and skin-prick testing with common allergens are occasionally performed to confirm the diagnosis of atopic eczema. Treatment of eczema is mainly topical, except in more severe cases, when systemic steroids and immunosuppressants are used. Therapies include the following:
- Emollients: moisturize dry skin and reduce itching.
- Topical steroids: anti-inflammatory agents.
- Topical antibiotics or antiseptics: for infected eczema.
- Oral antihistamine: reduces itching.
- Cyclosporine: resistant cases may require immunosuppression.

Allergic rhinitis

Nasal congestion, watery nasal discharge, and sneezing occur after exposure to allergen. The most common allergens are grass, flower, weed or tree pollens, which cause a seasonal rhinitis (hay fever), and house-dust-mite feces, which can cause a more perennial rhinitis. Allergic attacks usually last for a few hours and are often accompanied by smarting and watering of the eyes. Skin-prick tests can identify the allergen.

Treatment is with antihistamines, steroids (nasal or ocular), or mast-cell stabilizers such as sodium cromoglycate. Avoidance of allergens is advised but is often difficult.

Anaphylaxis

Anaphylaxis is a medical emergency and can be fatal. However, it is rapidly reversible if treated properly. A systemic response to an allergen that is either intravenous or rapidly absorbed can cause tracheal occlusion and shock. Many allergens can cause anaphylaxis, but more common causes include drugs, bee stings, and peanuts. The signs of anaphylaxis are principally those of shock. Signs include the following:

- Hypotension with tachycardia.
- Warm peripheral temperature.
- Signs of airway obstruction.
- Laryngeal and facial edema and urticaria (often seen).

The initial management of anaphylaxis is resuscitation. Allergens should be removed if possible (e.g., stop drug infusion), and the patient should be given high-flow oxygen. Epinephrine should be given intramuscularly and repeated after 5 minutes if there is no improvement. Epinephrine should be given intravenously only in life-threatening profound shock. Fluids might be needed for patients in shock, and a β_2-adrenoreceptor agonist can be used to reverse bronchospasm. People who have had anaphylactic reactions often carry epinephrine with them so that it can be administered rapidly in an emergency. Steroids and antihistamines act too slowly to be effective in anaphylaxis.

Etiology of atopy (allergy)

Genetic and environmental factors contribute to determining whether an individual manifests an atopic (Th2 predominant, IgE) or immune (Th1 predominant, IgG) reaction to an antigen. The high prevalence of atopic disease (20%) in developed countries compared to developing countries has resulted in the proposal of a "hygiene hypothesis" to explain the disparity. Simply stated, individuals living in a more "hygienic" (Western) environment that precludes early and extensive antigen exposure leads to a higher likelihood of Th2 response to antigens.

 The hygiene hypothesis is proposed to account for the much greater incidence of allergy in Western nations.

The following observations in general support the hygiene hypothesis:
1. Th1 response is more common when:
- Older siblings are present.
- There is early exposure to care in a group setting.
- There is a high risk of tuberculosis, measles, or hepatitis A exposure.
- Children live in a rural environment.

2. Th2 response is more common when:
- There is frequent and widespread use of antibiotics.
- Children live in an urban environment.
- Children consume a "Western-style" diet.

Management of allergic disease

Allergic complaints constitute a significant proportion of visits to physicians' offices. It is common for mild allergic problems to be managed by pharmacologic blocking of mediators of IgE-mediated reactions (type 1 hypersensitivity). Agents commonly used include the following:
- Antihistamines.
- Antileukotrienes.
- Anti-inflammatory agents, especially topical or inhaled cortiocosteroids.

Allergen avoidance can be effective for food and drug allergies, but respiratory allergies are less easily managed in this manner. Especially in more severe allergic conditions, desensitization is often undertaken. Desensitization involves repeated injection of dilute solutions of allergen with slow increase of the allergen dosage (Fig. 11.2).

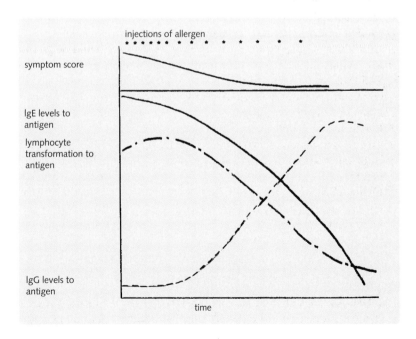

Fig. 11.2 Changes over time with desensitization therapy.

71

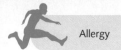

Symptomatic treatment is used for mild allergy; desensitization is used for more severe allergy.

Desensitization results in:
- Downregulation of Th2 cells and upregulation of Th1 cells and other regulatory T cells.
- Increased release of cytokines that favor antigen hyporesponsiveness (IL-10 and TNF-β).
- Increasing titers of IgG compete for or block the specific allergen one is injecting.

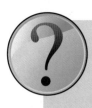

- Define asthma, and list its most common symptoms.
- List the mechanisms that cause the symptoms in asthma.
- Explain how asthma is diagnosed and treated.
- Define atopic eczema, and list its most common symptoms.
- Explain how atopic eczema is diagnosed and treated.
- Define allergic rhinitis, and list its most common symptoms.
- Explain how allergic rhinitis is diagnosed and treated.
- Define anaphylaxis, and list its most common causes.
- Explain how anaphylaxis is treated.
- Explain the hygiene hypothesis.
- Summarize the management of allergic disease.

12. Autoimmunity

Prevention of autoimmunity

Autoimmunity is a state in which the body exhibits immunologic reactivity to itself. "Self-tolerance" is the generic term given to the mechanisms by which T and B cells are prevented from responding to self. Because T and B cells randomly recombine the genes for their receptors, there is a risk of producing receptors that will react with self-antigen. These cells must be eliminated to make the host tolerant to itself.

Central tolerance
Central tolerance is by negative selection—early clonal deletion. T cells (in the thymus) and B cells (in the bone marrow) are eliminated if they are self-reactive. Central tolerance is not complete. Only the most self-reactive lymphocytes are deleted, ensuring that a wide lymphocyte repertoire is maintained.

Peripheral tolerance
In the periphery, self-antigens do not generally elicit an immune response. Several mechanisms prevent self-reactive T cells from causing autoimmune disease, including the following:

- Lack of the costimulatory molecules required for T-cell activation (e.g., cells expressing self-antigen do not express CD-40 or CD-28).
- Sequestration of the antigen behind a physical barrier (e.g., the testis).
- Lack of antigen presentation.
- T cells entering immune-privileged sites undergo apoptosis (via Fas, transforming growth factor [TGF]-β, or IL-10). Immune-privileged sites include the brain, testis, and anterior chamber of the eye.
- A negative feedback system (cytotoxic T lymphocyte antigen 4) prevents overstimulation of an immune response.

Immune regulation
Response to self-antigen can also be regulated by a population of T cells producing suppressive cytokines. Regulatory T cells inhibit responses of other T cells through mechanisms that are as yet poorly understood.

Causes of autoimmunity—breakdown of tolerance

If tolerance breaks down, autoimmunity can develop. Tolerance can break down in the thymus (usually for genetic reasons) or in the periphery (usually as a result of environmental factors such as infection). Autoimmunity is multifactorial; a defect in at least one of the regulatory mechanisms is required before disease develops.

Role of human leukocyte antigen (HLA)—genetic predisposition
Many autoimmune diseases have a familial component. The HLA haplotype is the main identified genetic factor. The haplotype can influence susceptibility to developing autoimmunity via molecular mimicry. Certain HLA alleles are linked to specific autoimmune processes (e.g., HLA-DR4 in rheumatoid arthritis). However, a certain HLA haplotype does not automatically result in the development of an autoimmune disease; 95% of patients with ankylosing spondylitis have HLA-B27, but only 5% of the population with HLA-B27 have ankylosing spondylitis.

Release of sequestered antigens
Sequestered antigens are not seen by the developing immune system; therefore, they are not deleted centrally. Tissue trauma can release previously sequestered antigen into the circulation, and an immune response can develop as a consequence.

Role of infection—molecular mimicry
Certain bacteria and viruses possess antigens that resemble sequestered host-cell components, and infection with these can generate an immune response against self. An example of molecular mimicry is cross-reactivity between heart muscle and streptococcal antigens, leading to rheumatic fever. This is short lived and reversible.

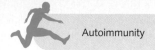

Role of infection—polyclonal activation

Some viral infections are able to activate B cells in a nonspecific fashion. This results in the proliferation of several B cell clones, which can produce autoreactive autoantibody.

Role of HLA—inappropriate MHC expression

Upregulation of MHC class II molecules can result in activation of autoreactive T cells. Healthy β cells in the islets of Langerhans have been shown to express low levels of class I and II MHC molecules, whereas cells in individuals with insulin-dependent diabetes mellitus (IDDM) express high levels of both.

Mechanisms of autoimmunity

Autoimmune conditions result from type II (antibody-mediated), type III (immune complex-mediated), and type IV (cell-mediated) immune reactions.

Type II mechanism autoimmune disease

Autoantibodies develop that directly interact with antigens on cell surfaces. This interaction can take many forms. If the antibody interaction is with a receptor that governs cells' function, it can stimulate or block the cell function (antireceptor antibody disease). If the antibody that binds to the cell surface antigen acts to opsonize the cell, it can lead to cell destruction either by monocyte phagocytosis or complement activation and lysis (destructive antibody disease). Type II mechanism autoimmune diseases usually involve only one organ or tissue.

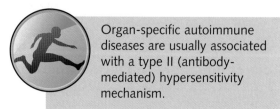

Organ-specific autoimmune diseases are usually associated with a type II (antibody-mediated) hypersensitivity mechanism.

The mechanism of antireceptor autoimmune disease is summarized in Fig. 12.1.

Examples of antireceptor autoimmune disease include the following:

- Graves' disease: associated with an antibody directed against the receptor for thyroid-stimulating hormone (TSH), resulting in release of T_4 and hyperthyroidism.
- Myasthenia gravis: associated with an antibody directed against the acetylcholine receptor, resulting in muscle weakness.

The mechanism of destructive antibody autoimmune disease is summarized in Fig. 12.2.

Examples of destructive antibody autoimmune disease include the following:

- Autoimmune hemolytic anemia: antibody directed against the Rh blood group or I blood group, which results in destruction of red blood cells in the spleen or by complement lysis.
- Autoimmune thrombocytopenia purpura: antibody directed against platelet integrin or glycoprotein IIb/IIa, which results in destruction of platelets in the spleen and bleeding.
- Pemphigus vulgaris: antibody directed against epidermal cadherin, which results in skin blistering.
- Goodpasture syndrome: antibody directed against type IV collagen, which results in basement membrane disruption and bleeding.

A special form of type II mechanism autoimmune disease results when autoantibodies arise against antigens in the cytoplasm of neutrophils. These

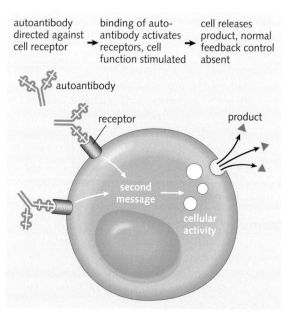

Fig. 12.1 Mechanism of antireceptor autoimmune disease.

antineutrophil cytoplasmic antibodies (ANCA) result in systemic vasculitis syndromes. Antibodies to myeloperoxidase (p-ANCA) lead to a necrotizing inflammation of medium-sized arteries known as polyarteritis nodosa. Antibodies to proteinase-3 (c-ANCA) lead to granulomatous arteritis, characteristically in the respiratory tract and kidney, known as Wegener granulomatosis. These antibodies are defined by indirect immunofluorescence testing using fixed neutrophils.

Type III mechanism autoimmune disease

In type III mechanism autoimmune disease, circulating immune complexes deposit in the capillaries of a variety of tissues, activate complement, and lead to an inflammatory reaction. Since circulating immune complexes are key to their pathogenesis; type III mechanism autoimmune diseases are usually systemic autoimmune diseases.

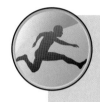

Systemic autoimmune diseases are frequently associated with a type III (immune complex-mediated) hypersensitivity mechanism.

It is a common practice to screen the serum of patients with suspected immune complex diseases by indirect immunofluorescence for antigens that bind to the nucleus in frozen sections of normal tissue (antinuclear antigens or ANA). Not only is the identification of an ANA useful in confirming systemic autoimmune disease, but the pattern of the ANA staining of the nucleus suggests specific autoantibodies that can then be confirmed with specific ELISA testing. Fig. 12.3 shows the use of ANA screening.

Anti-ds DNA is characteristic of systemic lupus erythematosus (SLE), which also may exhibit a number of antihistone antibodies. The extractable

autoantibody directed against cell surface antigen ➡ binding of autoantibody activates complement ➡ cell is destroyed

autoantibody

target antigen

C1

C2

C4

membrane attack

Fig. 12.2 Mechanism of destructive antibody autoimmune disease.

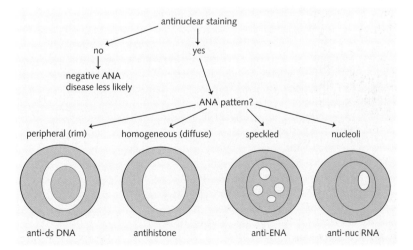

antinuclear staining

no → negative ANA disease less likely

yes → ANA pattern?

peripheral (rim)   homogeneous (diffuse)   speckled   nucleoli

anti-ds DNA   antihistone   anti-ENA   anti-nuc RNA

Fig. 12.3 Use of antinuclear antibody screening.

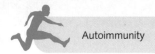
nuclear antigens (ENA) are seen in many systemic autoimmune diseases, including SLE (anti-SM), Sjögren syndrome (anti-SS-A and SS-B), mixed connective tissue disease (anti-RNP), and scleroderma (Scl-1). The antinucleolar RNA antibodies are seen in Raynaud's syndrome and scleroderma.

SLE is the classic type III mediated immune complex disease. Immune complexes are trapped in the microvasculature in multiple areas:

- Central nervous system (choroid plexus complexes): seizures, psychosis.
- Skin (D–E junction complexes): butterfly rash.
- Serositis (lining membrane complexes of lungs and heart): pleuritis, pericarditis, endocarditis.
- Spleen (activation, increased phagocytic activity): anemia, leukopenia, and thrombocytopenia.
- Kidney (glomerular complexes): glomerulonephritis.
- Joints (synovial complexes): arthritis.
- Lymph nodes (activation): lymphadenopathy.

Type IV mechanism autoimmune disease

The type IV mechanism autoimmune diseases result from autoimmune T-cell responses. Both T helper and T cytotoxic cells may be involved.

Examples of type IV mechanism autoimmune diseases are as follows:

- Type I diabetes mellitus: pancreatic islet cells are targeted.
- Polymyositis: striated muscle cells are targeted.
- Multiple sclerosis: myelin basic protein is targeted.
- Rheumatoid arthritis: synovial antigens are targeted (Figs. 12.4 and 12.5).

MHC-locus disease association

The chromosomal region where the MHC genes reside is highly polymorphic, has a very high density of genes, and it appears to contain a large number of genes that affect susceptibility to a number of conditions.

- Since MHC genes are associated with antigen presentation, it is reasonable that susceptibility or resistance to infectious agents could be linked to MHC types (i.e., some MHC antigen configurations interact more effectively with certain antigens). Recent studies have linked susceptibility and rapidity of progression of HIV infections with certain HLA antigens.
- Since MHC genes are important in mediation of the immune response, it is reasonable that autoimmune disease might be linked with HLA type. One of the longest-known and strongest links

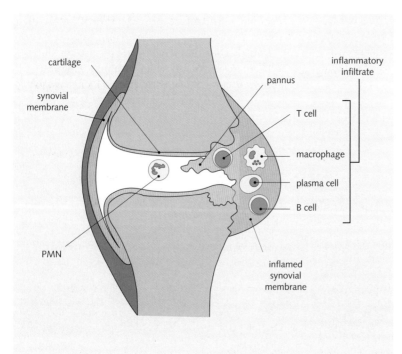

Fig. 12.4 Rheumatoid joint showing pannus formation and cartilage destruction. The synovial membrane is infiltrated by inflammatory cells and hypertrophies to form granulation tissue known as "pannus." This process eventually erodes the articular cartilage and bone. T cells and macrophages in the inflamed synovium secrete tumor necrosis factor (PMN, polymorphonuclear neutrophil).

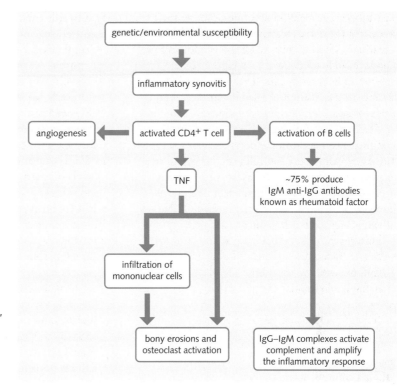

Fig. 12.5 Pathogenesis of rheumatoid arthritis (RA). Autoreactive CD4$^+$ T cells mediate the pathologic changes. Synovial T cells produce a number of cytokines, including tumor necrosis factor (TNF). These cytokines stimulate the acute-phase response, synovial inflammation, and bone erosion. Activation of B cells can result in the production of rheumatoid factor and immune complex formation.

between an HLA antigen and inflammatory disease is ankylosing spondylitis and HLA-B27 (Fig. 12.6).

Demonstration of disease to MHC-type linkage is complicated by two phenomena:

- MHC region susceptibility genes appear to demonstrate incomplete penetrance (i.e., the gene is present but not expressed).
- MHC region associations vary greatly between racial and ethnic groups (presumed to be due to long-term genetic reassortment).

Management of autoimmune disorders

A number of pharmacologic agents are available that affect T-cell function and are of potential value in controlling autoimmune disorders (these will be explored in greater detail when transplantation is discussed). Many autoimmune disorders are antibody mediated, and so removal of antibody and suppression of antibody production or activity are the most logical approaches to their management.

MHC loci associations with diseases	
Disease	**MHC association**
	Class I genes
Ankylosing spondylitis	HLA-B27
Graves disease	HLA-B8w35 or Bw36
Psoriasis	HLA-Cw6
HIV infection risk	HLA-Cw7
Rapid HIV progression	HLA-B7 and HLA-B35
	Class II genes
Rheumatoid arthritis	HLA-DR4 or DR1
SLE	HLA-DR2 or DR3
Celiac disease	HLA-DR3, DQA1
Phemphigus vulgaris	HLA-DR6
Type 1 diabetes mellitus	HLA-DR4, DQB1
Multiple sclerosis	HLA-DR2, DQB1
Hashimoto thyroiditis	HLA-DR5 or DR3

Fig. 12.6 MHC loci associations with diseases.

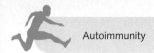

Antibody can be removed from the plasma by a process of plasmapheresis. Using a specially modified centrifuge, blood is anticoagulated, removed from the body, and centrifuged to separate red cells and plasma. Then the red cells, usually diluted in albumin, are reinfused. Although this is rapidly effective and used in acute situations, it is not a long-term solution.

Infusion of high doses of intravenous immunoglobulin has been found to be useful in a number of autoimmune diseases. Autoimmune diseases in which controlled clinical trials have demonstrated the efficacy of immunoglobulin infusions include the following:

- Immune thrombocytopenic purpura.
- Myasthenia gravis.
- ANCA-mediated vasculitis.
- Multiple sclerosis.

The mechanism by which infusion of high-dose immunoglobulin works is complex and involves effects on multiple elements of the immune response:

- **Fc receptor effects.** The Fc portions of the infused immunoglobulins bind to and result in a blockage of Fc receptors on macrophages, preventing them from attaching to and engulfing IgG coasted cells or platelets.

- **Anti-inflammatory effects.** Large amounts of infused IgG prevent generation of the complement membrane attack complex by binding C3b and C4b and preventing the deposition of these activated components on cell surfaces. High levels of infused IgG can also bind to antigen or complement components in immune complexes, lessening their ability to further activate complement and speeding the complex clearance. It also appears that high IgG levels downregulate endothelial cell-activation molecules.

- **Effects on B cells and autoantibodies.** As noted in the discussion of normal regulation of immune system, anti-idiotype antibodies are provided in the high dose infused immunoglobulins, and they can act to neutralize autoantibodies by binding to the active sites and effect B-cell activity by blocking surface antigen receptor sites. There is also some suggestion that anti-idiotype antigens to T-cell receptors can modulate their function.

- **Effects on cell growth.** Evidence suggests that high levels of infused immunoglobulin result in inhibition of lymphocyte proliferation, again probably via receptor blockage, and may result in increased lymphocyte apoptosis.

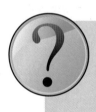

- How does the body prevent self-reactive lymphocytes from causing autoimmune disease?
- What role do infection and human leukocyte antigen (HLA) molecules play in autoimmune disease?
- What causes systemic lupus erythematosus? What are the major symptoms?
- What pathologic processes occur in rheumatoid arthritis?
- Compare and contrast Hashimoto's thyroiditis and Graves' disease.
- How is insulin-dependent (type 1) diabetes mellitus related to autoimmunity?

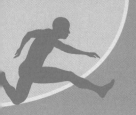

13. Anti-Inflammatory Drugs

Anti-inflammatory drugs are used commonly for the treatment of a variety of conditions. Different types of anti-inflammatory drugs are available, including the following:

- Steroids.
- Nonsteroidal anti-inflammatory drugs.
- Inhibitors of leukotriene function.
- Tumor necrosis factor antagonists.

Steroids

The adrenal cortex releases several steroid hormones into the circulation. Glucocorticoids affect carbohydrate and protein metabolism, but also have effects on the immune system, acting as immunosuppressive and anti-inflammatory agents. Several glucocorticoids are available therapeutically, including the following:

- Hydrocortisone: can be given intravenously in status asthmaticus or topically for inflammatory skin conditions.
- Prednisolone: oral preparations given in many inflammatory or allergic conditions.
- Beclomethasone: used as an aerosol in asthma or topically for eczema.

Conditions commonly treated with steroids include these:

- Inflammatory bowel disease.
- Allergic conditions (e.g., asthma).
- Severe inflammatory skin conditions.
- Severe inflammatory rheumatologic conditions.

Steroids act by entering cells, particularly macrophages, where they bind receptors and stimulate the transcription of hundreds of genes. Suppression of inflammation occurs by a variety of mechanisms:

- Reduction in the number of circulating lymphocytes and macrophages.
- Inhibition of phospholipase A2 and therefore the formation of proinflammatory arachidonic acid metabolites.
- Inhibition of complement.

Adverse effects and contraindications

Glucocorticoids cause many adverse effects at the high doses required to produce an anti-inflammatory effect. The clinical features are similar to those seen in Cushing's syndrome, and the adverse effects are shown in Fig. 13.1. Steroids are contraindicated if there is evidence of systemic infection. Long-term high-dose steroid therapy is usually avoided.

Adverse effects of glucocorticoids	
Body system	**Symptoms**
Gastrointestinal	Dyspepsia, nausea, peptic ulceration, abdominal distension, acute pancreatitis, esophageal ulceration, candidiasis
Musculoskeletal	Proximal myopathy, osteoporosis, avascular osteonecrosis
Endocrine	Adrenal suppression, menstrual irregularities, hirsutism, weight gain, negative nitrogen and calcium balance, increased appetite, increased susceptibility to infection
Neuropsychiatric	Euphoria, psychological dependence, depression, insomnia, aggravation of epilepsy, psychosis
Ophthalmic	Glaucoma, papilloedema, cataracts
Skin	Impaired wound healing, atrophy, easy bruising, striae, telangiectasia, acne

Fig. 13.1 The adverse effects of glucocorticoids.

Nonsteroidal anti-inflammatory drugs (NSAIDs)

NASIDs include a large number of chemically diverse drugs that inhibit cyclo-oxygenase (COX) and hence interfere with prostaglandin production. They are not only anti-inflammatory but also have some analgesic effects. Acetylsalicylic acid (aspirin) is the oldest example of this class of drugs, which includes indomethacin, ibuprofen, and the more recently developed COX-2 inhibitors. The less specific (older) drugs are associated with significant gastrointestinal side effects. Newer COX-2 inhibitors appear to have cardiovascular side effects.

Inhibitors of leukotriene function (LtIs)

Leukotrienes are also arachidonic acid (AA)-derived mediators of inflammation. Leukotriene-inhibiting (LtI) drugs include leukotriene-receptor antagonists (montelukast) and inhibitors of 5-lipoxygenase (zileuton), which catalyze the formation of leukotrienes from AA. These drugs are most commonly used in asthma. They have relatively few side effects, probably due to the fact that production of leukotrienes is predominantly limited to sites of inflammation.

Fig. 13.2 illustrates the site of action of corticosteroids, NSAIDs, and LtIs.

Tumor necrosis factor (TNF) antagonists

TNF-α is a major inflammatory cytokine important in the pathogenesis of several autoimmune and chronic inflammatory disorders. Blockage of the effect of TNF-α has been shown useful in the management of such conditions. Two strategies have been used:

- Development of synthetic soluble TNF-receptor proteins that bind to the cytokine, preventing it from interacting with it cellular receptors (etanercept).
- Development of monoclonal antibodies directed against TNF-α (infliximab, adalimumab, anakinra). The antibody binds with soluble and membrane-bound TNF-α and neutralizes it or lyses the cells expressing it on their surfaces.

Both of these types of TNF-α antagonists have been shown to be useful in rheumatoid arthritis and inflammatory bowel disease. These agents are not without side effects, which include the following:

- Risk of serious infection.
- Reactivation of occult tuberculosis.
- Increased incidence of lymphoma.
- Allergic reactions: antibodies may form to the antagonists.

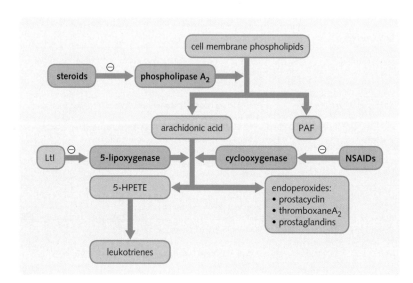

Fig. 13.2 The actions of nonsteroidal anti-inflammatory drugs (NSAIDs) and leukotriene-inhibiting (LtI) drugs in arachidonic acid metabolism (PAF, platelet-activating factor).

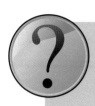

- What types of drugs are used to reduce inflammation?
- What conditions are commonly treated with steroids?
- By what mechanisms do steroid reduce inflammation?
- What are the contraindications to steroid use?
- How do NSAIDs and leukotriene inhibitors achieve their effects?

14. Transplantation

A transplant is the transfer of tissue from one individual to another. Blood transfusion is the most common "tissue transfer." Donor selection and testing for blood transfusion provide a good introduction to analogous processes in organ and stem-cell transplantation.

Blood transfusion

Red-cell antigens

The surfaces of red cells are covered with antigenic molecules. Over 400 different groups of antigens have been identified, although only some of these are clinically important in blood transfusion. Some red-cell antigens can be recognized by antibodies in the serum of a recipient of a blood transfusion and can cause an adverse reaction. Because these reactions can be severe and life threatening, it is important to identify the antigens and antibodies present in both donor and recipient blood.

ABO antigens

The ABO system consists of three allelic genes—A, B, and O—which code for sugar-residue transferase enzymes. The ABO antigen, known as the H antigen, is a glycoprotein or glycolipid with a terminal L-fructose.

- The O gene is amorphous; that is, it has no effect on antigenic structure and leaves antigen H unchanged.
- The group A gene-product adds N-acetyl galactosamine to the H antigen.
- The group B gene-product adds the sugar D-galactose (Fig. 14.1).

Inheritance of the three ABO alleles can lead to six different genotypes and four possible phenotypes (Fig. 14.2).

By 6 months of age, the immune system will have been exposed to A- and B-like antigens in intestinal bacteria and food substances. IgM antibodies develop against A and/or B antigens, unless these antigens are present on red cells. Transfused blood must be ABO-compatible with the recipient's blood; otherwise, recipient antibody will cause agglutination and hemolysis of the transfused cells. For example, if group A red cells are given to a group O recipient, anti-A antibodies in the recipient's serum will destroy the donor cells.

Ideally, ABO-identical blood is used; however, if this is not possible, compatible blood can be used. Blood cells of group O are not affected by anti-A or anti-B antibodies and can therefore be given to patients of any blood group. Consequently, blood group O is referred to as the universal donor. Conversely, AB individuals are universal recipients because they do not possess anti-ABO antibodies and can receive blood of any ABO type.

Rhesus antigens

Rhesus (Rh) antigens are good immunogens, and the antibodies generated are clinically important. They

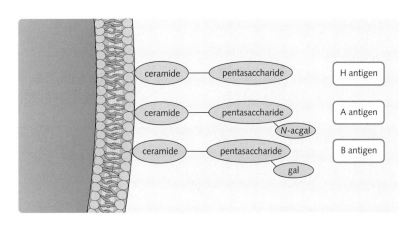

Fig. 14.1 ABO antigens (N-acgal, N-acetylgalactosamine; gal, galactose).

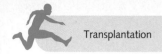

are known as C, D, and E, but the D antigen is the most important clinically. It is the D antigen that is referred to when someone is described as "Rh-positive" or "Rh-negative." The rhesus locus on chromosome 1 consists of two closely linked genes, RhD and RhCE, which are inherited together. RhD encodes the D antigen; "d" denotes the absence of D antigen (Fig. 14.3). The gene RhCE encodes antigens named C, c, E, and e. Note that "c" and "e" are real antigens and not just the absence of an antigen, like "d." Alternate gene splicing of RhCE produces two proteins.

D antigen is the strongest immunogen. Rh-positive individuals are DD or Dd, Rh-negative individuals are dd. Approximately 85% of Caucasians are Rh-positive, and 15% are Rh-negative.

Anti-D antibodies are generated only when an Rh-negative individual is exposed to Rh-positive red cells following transfusion or pregnancy. All anti-D antibodies are IgG. Approximately 70% of Rh-negative individuals produce anti-D antibodies after receiving Rh-positive blood, and they could develop transfusion reactions when retransfused with Rh-positive blood.

Cross-matching for blood transfusion

In order to ensure that red blood cells are safe for transfusion, red cells of an appropriate type must be selected (typing). In addition, the patient's serum must be reacted with screening cells and the red cells to be transfused to determine whether unexpected antibodies are present in the serum (screening and cross-matching).

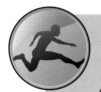

Blood transfusion is the most common tissue transplant. To ensure that no immune reaction occurs, careful matching of donor antigen and recipient antibodies is needed.

Blood typing

The donor's cells are reacted with antibodies from animals against A and B antigens. If the A or B antigen is present on the surface of the donor cells, the antibodies will attach, causing the cells to agglutinate. A "back-type" can also be performed. The donor's serum is reacted against known A and B cells to ensure that the appropriate naturally occurring antibodies are present, confirming the direct (forward) type. Red cells are Rh (D)-typed using anti-D antibodies:

- O red cells can be given to O, A, B, or AB recipients.
- A red cells can be given to A or AB recipients.
- B red cells can be given to B or AB recipients.
- AB red cells can be given only to AB recipients.
- Rh (D)-positive cells can be transfused only to Rh-positive individuals.
- Rh (D)-negative cells can be transfused to either Rh-positive or Rh-negative individuals.

Screening and cross-matching

The recipient's serum is incubated with a panel of O cells that express the majority of known red cell antigens and with the red cells of the potential donor unit. If agglutination occurs, then the unexpected antigen is identified, and only red cells that lack that antigen are used for transfusion. To be sure that no unexpected antibody is present in the donor's serum, a second step to detect it is undertaken. After a

ABO blood groups		
Phenotype/red cell antigens	Genotype	Antibodies
O	OO	Anti-A and Anti-B
A	AO or AA	Anti-B
B	BO or BB	Anti-A
AB	AB	None

Fig. 14.2 ABO blood groups.

Rhesus genotypes	
CDE genotype	RhD
cde/cde	Negative
CDe/cde	Positive
CDe/CDe	Positive
cDE/cde	Positive
CDe/cDE	Positive
cDE/cDE	Positive
Others	Most are positive

Fig. 14.3 Rhesus genotypes.

period of incubation in recipient serum, the red cells are washed and then reacted with antibody directed against human immunoglobulin. Evidence of both macroscopic and microscopic agglutination is sought (antiglobulin or Coombs' test). Only red cells that test negative for antiglobulin are transfused.

Hemolytic transfusion reactions

If red cells are transfused that have antigens on their surface to which the recipient has antibodies in the serum, the red cells are destroyed. Cells mismatched for ABO result in rapid destruction of the red cells and a potentially fatal systemic immune reaction that is associated with extensive mediator activation.

Solid organ and stem-cell transplantation

Common types of solid organ and stem-cell transplantation performed today are summarized in Fig. 14.4.

Unless the donor and recipient are immunologically identical, the recipient will mount a rejection response against "foreign" antigens expressed by the graft. The most important graft antigens responsible for an immune response in the recipient are the MHC molecules. However, even when the donor and recipient are genetically identical at the MHC loci, graft rejection can occur

Autologous grafts are grafts moved from one part of the body to another (e.g., skin grafts).
Syngeneic grafts are between genetically identical individuals (e.g., monozygotic twins).
Allogeneic grafts are between individuals of the same species.
Xenogeneic grafts are between different species.

due to differences at other loci, which encode minor histocompatibility antigens. A rejection response can lead to loss of a graft. There are three types of graft rejection (Fig. 14.5):

- Hyperacute.
- Acute cellular.
- Chronic.

Graft versus host disease

The characteristics of graft versus host disease are summarized in Fig. 14.6.

Stem cells can be obtained from bone marrow, from blood after mobilization by steroids and growth factor, and from umbilical cord blood (which has a high level of stems cells that may be less prone to

Common transplants	
Transplant	**Notes**
Kidney	Live or cadaveric donor; the fewer the MHC mismatches, the greater the success rate; must be ABO compatible
Heart	Matching is beneficial, but often time is a more pressing concern
Liver	No evidence to suggest that matching affects graft survival; rejection less aggressive than for other organs
Skin graft	Most grafts are autologous, but allografts can be used to protect burn patients
Corneal graft	Matching (class II MHC) is required only if a previous graft was vascularized
Stem cell	Host-versus-graft (HVG) or graft-versus-host (GVH) responses possible. The transplant must be well matched and antirejection therapy used. Host immune cells are destroyed by irradiation prior to transplant (avoids HVG). T cells are depleted from the graft (avoids GVH) using monoclonal antibody and complement

Fig. 14.4 Common transplants.

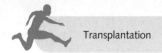

Patterns of graft rejection		
Type	Mechanism	Prevention
Hyperacute (minutes–hours)	Pre-existing antidonor antibodies	Perform cross-match of donor cells and recipient's serum, check for ABO compatibility
Acute cellular (days–weeks)	T cell mediated	HLA matching of donor and recipient, antirejection therapy
Chronic (months–years)	Unclear	HLA matching

Fig. 14.5 Patterns of graft rejection (HLA, human leukocyte antigen).

Characteristics of graft vs. host disease		
Characteristic	Acute	Chronic
Onset	Early	Late
Systems affected most commonly	Skin, GI	Skin, lung
Mechanism	T-cell response	Immunoglobulins
Pathology	Cellular infiltrate and epithelial cell damage	Vascular damage and fibrosis
Treatment	Immunosuppression	None

Fig. 14.6 Characteristics of graft versus host disease.

cause graft versus host disease). The best HLA matches are generally found in first-degree relatives, although unrelated marrow donor registries exist. Chances of rejection and severe graft versus host disease are more common with unrelated donor transplants, probably because even if HLA-A, HLA-B, and HLA-D matches are found, it is much less likely that linked minor HLA antigens will also be the same.

Antirejection therapy

Immunosuppressive drugs are used to prevent and treat rejection (predominantly cellular rejection). Drugs that are used to prevent rejection inhibit lymphocyte activation and proliferation or destroy lymphoid cells. Common antirejection drugs are:

- **Early acting drugs:** bind to immunophilins, forming a complex that binds to the phosphatase calcineurin and inhibits the calcineurin-catalyzed dephosphorylation essential to activate nuclear factors of T cells. Examples include cyclosporine and tacrolimus.
- **Late-acting drugs:** antimetabolite agents that interfere with DNA metabolism and hence cell proliferation. Examples include azathioprine and mycophenolate.
- **Drugs acting both early and late:** prednisone (corticosteroids).
- **Monoclonal antibodies:** anti-C3 antibodies destroy T cells, whereas anti-IL-2 receptor antibodies block T-cell activation.

In many transplant centers, a sequence of immunosuppressive drugs is used. At the time of transplant (induction), monoclonal antibodies and high-dose steroids are used to allow initial engraftment. Combinations of an early acting and late-acting drug are then used for maintenance therapy. If cellular rejection occurs, monoclonal antibodies are often used to attempt to control it.

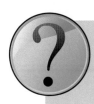

- Why are typing and cross-matching needed before a blood transfusion?
- How are typing and cross-matching performed?
- What is graft versus host disease?
- Why are transplanted organs rejected?
- What steps can be taken to prevent rejection of transplanted organs?

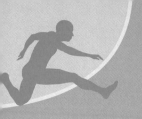

15. Pregnancy and Immune-Mediated Diseases of the Fetus and Newborn

Immunology of pregnancy

In view of the previous discussion about transplantation and the need for immunosuppression for allograft survival, the immunologic events involved in pregnancy, during which a haplo-nonidentical fetus develops successfully within the uterus, is of interest. Several immunologic aspects of pregnancy will be discussed.

Fertilization is dependent on immune mechanisms. The fusion step of sperm-ova fertilization is mediated by the interaction of MHC class II molecules on the posterior sperm head and CD4/p56 Lck molecules on the ova membrane. This fact explains why species specificity is required for fertilization. Antibodies against sperm antigens are known to be associated with infertility.

Trophoblasts (cells that cover the placental villi and are at the maternal–fetal interface) have unique characteristics that modulate the maternal immune response:

- Trophoblasts do not demonstrate usual HLA antigens associated with classic recognition of nonself (HLA-A, -B, and -D). Rather, they demonstrate rarely expressed HLA antigens (HLA-C, -E, and -G), which bind to NK cell inhibitory receptors. NK cells constitute 60–70% of immunologically active cells in the deciduus.
- Trophoblasts express large amounts of complement control proteins on their surfaces (decay-activating factor or DAF), which is assumed to minimize complement cascade activity.
- Trophoblasts express an enzyme, indolamine 2- to 3-dioxygenase (IDO), which catabolizes tryptophane to metabolites that act to suppress T-cell activation in the deciduus. Pharmacologic blockade of IDO results in prompt abortion.

The trophoblast cells that cover the surface of the placenta in contact with the mother play a major role in allowing pregnancy to occur without an immunologic reaction to the fetus.

Decidual immune cells do respond to the presence of a conceptus, and this response is important to the appropriate progression of a pregnancy. NK cells secrete growth factors and cytokines that control trophoblastic invasion and play a role in decidual vascular remodeling.

Microchimerism induced by small numbers of fetal cells that reach the maternal circulation may under some circumstances induce peripheral tolerance by clonal deletion.

The immunologic phenomenon associated with pregnancy influence other maternal immune functions:

- Cell-mediated autoimmune diseases such as rheumatoid arthritis tend to improve during pregnancy.
- Antibody-mediated processes such as SLE are exacerbated by pregnancy.
- Immunologic processes appear to contribute to infertility and unexplained recurrent early abortion.
- Patients with antiphospholipid syndrome have a significantly increased risk of infertility and early abortion. Treatment of the condition by aspirin and heparin greatly improves outcome.
- More than half of women with unexplained recurrent abortions produce an embryotoxin in culture supernatants when their blood mononuclear cells are activated by trophoblastic tissue.
- Infusion of paternal leukocytes (to induce tolerance) benefits 10% of couples with recurrent unexplained pregnancy losses.

Immune-mediated diseases of the fetus and newborn

Fetuses have T-cell function by 20 weeks of gestation and can produce antibodies *in utero* if stimulated. Other than cases of blood-borne infection transmitted via the mother (e.g., cytomegalovirus, toxoplasmosis, rubella), fetuses generally do not produce antibodies (hence the utility of measuring neonatal IgM levels to screen for neonatal infection).

Passive antibody transfer across the placenta is the major source of antibody in the plasma of fetuses and neonates. Hence, if the maternal plasma contains antibodies that can injure the fetus, disease can result. Two types of syndromes are recognized:

- Passive transfer of autoantibodies, resulting in a disease state in the fetus.
- Passive transfer of antibodies directed against antigens in the fetus that the mother does not share (alloimmune) disease.

Passage of maternal antibodies across the placenta can result in disease in the fetus and newborn.

Passive transfer of autoantibodies

A mother with an autoimmune disease may have mild disease or may have been treated for the condition, but the antibodies persist in her serum and, when transferred across the placenta, cause injury the fetus. Fig. 15.1 gives examples of such conditions.

Alloimmune conditions

The alloimmune conditions are associated with the antibodies directed against fetal antigens that the mother lacks. The antibodies are invariably directed against blood cells or platelets. This occurs because sensitization is assumed to arise by fetal–maternal hemorrhages, which expose the mother to the foreign antigen.

Hemolytic disease of the newborn (HDN)

Red blood cell antigens enter the circulation of the mother, usually during the third trimester or at birth. The foreign red cell antigen stimulates a maternal immune response, and in subsequent pregnancies, when passive antibody transfer occurs, red cell hemolysis and fetal anemia result. Anti-D, because of its immunogenicity, has been the most common cause of HDN, but any of the other blood group antigens that can induce an IgG response can be responsible. HDN can be detected by monitoring amniotic fluid for increases in bilirubin levels in pregnancies where the mother's antibody screen demonstrates antibodies to an antigen that the father can transmit.

Anti-D HDN is now prevented by the administration of anti-D antibodies to anti-D negative mothers, usually at 28 weeks of gestation and at birth. The injected anti-D binds to any fetal D-positive cells that have gained access to the maternal circulation, causing them to be removed by the reticuloendothelial system before the mother can be sensitized.

Once an individual is sensitized to a blood group antigen, all future pregnancies with fetuses that bear that antigen will be affected, usually with increasingly severe disease. Once a mother is

Fetal diseases caused by passive transfer of autoantibodies		
Disease	**Autoantibody**	**Fetal condition**
Graves disease	Anti TSH receptor	Hyperthyroidism
Immune thrombocytopenic purpura (ITP)	Antiplatelet antibody	Hemorrhage Low platelet count
Systemic lupus vulgaris	Anti-Ro antibodies Anti-La antibodies	Rash Congenital heart block
Pemphigus vulgaris	Antidesmoglein 3	Blistering rash
Myasthenia gravis	Antiacetylcholine receptor	Hypotonia Weakness

Fig. 15.1 Fetal diseases caused by passive transfer of autoantibodies.

sensitized, procedures to remove maternal antibody (plasmapheresis) or fetal umbilical cord puncture and transfusion of red cells compatible with both mother and fetus can be used in an attempt to preserve the pregnancy.

Fetal alloimmune thrombocytopenia (FAP)

In FAP, the maternal serum usually contains antibodies to human platelet antigen A1 (HPA-1). It is assumed that sensitization occurs from fetal–maternal hemorrhage, but FAP often affects first pregnancies. Since platelet antibodies are not screened for, most cases are diagnosed when the newborn shows bruising and low platelet counts. Intracerebral hemorrhage is the most feared complication and can occur both *in utero* and after birth. Since more than 90% of individuals are HPA-1 positive, all pregnancies of women with known anti-HPA-1 are monitored by performing umbilical cord puncture to obtain platelet counts. If a fetus is affected, efforts to remove maternal antibody or *in utero* platelet transfusions (usually using the mother as the source of the platelets) can be undertaken.

Fetal alloimmune neutropenia (FAN)

FAN is the least serious of the alloimmune conditions, because it results in only a short period of increased risk of infection during the immediate postdelivery period. It is usually due to antibodies to human neutrophil antigen A1 (HNA-1). Recognition of FAN is important, as it can be confused with the neutropenia associated with overwhelming infection.

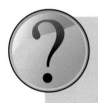

- How do trophoblasts allow pregnancy to occur without an immunologic reaction to the fetus?
- What other factors modulate the maternal immune response during pregnancy?
- What two types of syndromes may result in immune-mediated disease in the fetus or newborn? Give examples of each.

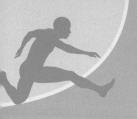
Leukemias

Leukemias are a group of disorders characterized by accumulation of abnormal blood cells in bone marrow. They are clonal disorders; that is, they result from successive uncontrolled divisions of a single cell. The leukemic "blast" cells are nonfunctional and replace normal bone marrow, encroaching on normal hematopoietic cell development. This leads to the following:

- Anemia.
- Neutropenia.
- Thrombocytopenia.

Many symptoms of leukemia are due to organ infiltration by leukemic cells. Organs that are commonly involved include the following:

- Bones.
- Lymph nodes.
- Liver and spleen (may also be involved by extramedullary hematopoiesis).
- Skin.
- Central nervous system.

Classification of leukemia is based on the following:

- Cell lineage (lymphoid or myeloid).
- Developmental stage of leukemic cells: acute leukemia involves proliferation of immature cells (blasts) and, untreated, is usually rapidly fatal; chronic leukemia involves more mature cells, and a more prolonged course is characteristic.

Acute myeloblastic leukemia

Acute myeloblastic leukemia (AML) is characterized by a rapidly progressive accumulation of primitive myeloblasts in bone marrow and peripheral blood. The incidence increases with age (median: 60 years),

with an average of 1 in 10,000 per year. The 5-year survival rate is about 50%. AML is associated with the following:

- Radiation exposure.
- Toxins: benzene, alkylating agents.
- Hereditary abnormalities (e.g., Down syndrome).
- Pre-existing hematologic disease: chronic myeloid leukemia (CML), myelodysplastic syndromes.

Patients are often acutely ill at presentation and can present with these symptoms:

- Anemia, malaise, sweats, weight loss.
- Infections (chest, mouth, skin).
- Bleeding.
- Skin infiltration.
- Leukostasis.

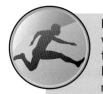

Leukostatic symptoms occur when white blood cells form thrombi in the heart, lungs, and brain. Symptoms include reduced consciousness, retinal hemorrhages, and pulmonary infiltrates.

Chromosome rearrangements have prognostic value: t(15;17), t(8;21), and inversion of 16 have better outcomes than monosomy 7.

AML is treated with combination chemotherapy and, in some cases, bone marrow transplantation. Thirty-five percent of people can be cured by chemotherapy alone, and the cure rate rises to 45% with bone marrow transplant. Survival is best in younger patients. The hematologic consequences of AML are treated to improve symptoms and outcome. This includes transfusions of red cells/platelets, leukapheresis to reduce blood viscosity, and the prevention/treatment of infection.

Chronic myeloid leukemia

CML, also known as chronic granulocytic leukemia, is a progressive accumulation of mature myeloid cells in blood and bone marrow. At presentation, the white cell count can be 300–500 × 109/L (normal levels are 4–11 × 109/L). It accounts for 20% of all leukemias. The average incidence is 1 in 100,000, peaking between 40 and 60 years of age. It is rare in children, and there is a slight male preponderance. Clinically, there are three phases of disease:

1. Chronic.
2. Accelerated.
3. Blast crisis (AML/ALL).

People normally present in the chronic phase following an incidental finding on a complete blood count or with constitutional (malaise, weight loss, sweats) or leukostatic symptoms. Some patients will quickly transform to an accelerated or blast crisis stage.

A disease marker, the Philadelphia chromosome, denoting a (9;22) translocation, is found in granulocytic, erythrocytic, and megakaryocytic precursor cells. This translocation fuses parts of two genes (BCR-ABL) to create an abnormal tyrosine kinase, which is thought to be involved in disease progression. A specific tyrosine kinase inhibitor is now available, which has improved outcome for these patients. Bone marrow transplantation is potentially curative.

Median survival is 5.5 years. Good prognostic factors include the following:
• Youth.
• Small spleen at presentation.
• Low white cell count at presentation.

Neoplasia of lymphoid origin

Acute lymphoblastic leukemia (ALL)
ALL accounts for 80% of all childhood leukemias but is rare in adults. The peak incidence occurs between 2 and 10 years of age. Presentation outside of this range confers a poorer prognosis. ALL is associated with:
• Radiation.
• Chemicals.
• Down syndrome.
• Fanconi's syndrome.

In 80% of cases, the blast cells are of B-cell origin. ALL is more responsive to combination chemotherapy than AML, and remission rates of 70% are attained. Cure rates are highest in females under

5 years old. The Philadelphia chromosome is seen in 10–20% of cases and is associated with a poor outcome.

Chronic lymphocytic leukemia (CLL)
CLL occurs most frequently in people over the age of 60 years (median age: 65 years) and accounts for 20–50% of all leukemias. It is twice as common in men as in women, with a total incidence of 3–4 per 10,000. CLL arises from a proliferation of neoplastic lymphoid cells (B cells), which infiltrate the marrow, lymph nodes, spleen, and liver. It is a slowly progressing, low-grade disorder. Symptoms seen in other leukemias are seen in 50% of CLL cases at diagnosis, and associated autoimmune hemolytic anemia is common.

On a blood film, leukemic cells resemble mature lymphocytes, although typical "smudge cells" are also seen. Disease transformation into acute leukemia does not occur. Median survival is 5–8 years, and treatment (chemotherapy or stem-cell transplantation) is usually aimed at limiting rather than curing the disease. Many elderly patients will die of an unrelated condition because of the slow nature of the disease.

Hairy cell leukemia
This condition causes a pancytopenia due to a monoclonal proliferation of a type of B cell with an irregular cytoplasmic outline. The number of "hairy" cells in the peripheral blood is highly variable; however, they are found in bone marrow. The peak incidence is 40–60 years of age, with males four times more likely than females to develop hairy cell leukemia. Treatment with 2-chlorodeoxyadenosine or deoxycoformycin causes remission in >90% of cases.

Malignant lymphomas

Lymphomas are a group of neoplastic disorders characterized by the proliferation of a primitive cell to produce a clonal expansion of lymphoid cells. They primarily involve the lymph nodes and extranodal lymphoid tissue (e.g., mucosal-associated lymphoid tissue [MALT] and spleen). Malignant lymphomas are divided into two categories:
• Non-Hodgkin's lymphoma.
• Hodgkin's disease (Hodgkin's lymphoma).

Although it is easy to think of leukemias as disease of the bone marrow and lymphomas as disease of the lymph nodes, remember that leukemic cells are found in the lymph nodes and that lymphoma cells commonly spread to the bone marrow and blood.

Non-Hodgkin's lymphomas

Non-Hodgkin's lymphomas (NHL) are a group of malignant diseases involving lymphoid cells. NHL is classified into low-, intermediate-, and high-grade disease in terms of clinical behavior (Fig. 16.1). Incidence of NHL rises with age and is more common in men than women. There are several etiological factors associated with NHL, including:

- Infections (e.g., Epstein-Barr virus and human T-cell lymphotrophic virus 1).
- Immunodeficiency (e.g., immunosuppressive therapy, HIV).
- Autoimmune disorders.
- Irradiation and carcinogens.
- Inherited disorders (e.g., ataxia telangiectasia, Fanconi's syndrome).

The incidence of NHL has increased since the 1970s, probably because of increases in the number of immunodeficient people. The features of NHL are outlined in Fig. 16.2.

Low-grade lymphomas

Follicle center cell lymphomas are the most common type. Low-grade disease has a benign course and responds to treatment. It is difficult to eradicate, and relapse is inevitable. Chemotherapy and monoclonal antibody therapy are often used. Survival is 7–10 years, and patients tend to die from resistant disease, infection, or transformation to a higher-grade lymphoma.

Intermediate-grade lymphomas

Mantle cell lymphomas are increasingly recognized as being intermediate grade. They do not respond well to treatment but progress rapidly (median survival: 3 years).

High-grade lymphomas

Large cell lymphomas are the most common. They respond well to treatment (40–50% long-term survival) if localized, but otherwise they are aggressive and rapidly progressive. The standard treatment regimen is known as CHOP (cyclophosphamide, adriamycin, vincristine, and prednisolone).

Hodgkin's disease

Hodgkin's disease (HD) characteristically affects young males in the third and fourth decades of life. There is a second peak of incidence in the elderly. Diagnosis requires the presence of pathognomonic Reed-Sternberg (RS) cells or derivatives, typically mixed with a variable inflammatory infiltrate.

REAL classification of non-Hodgkin's lymphoma		
Grade	B cell	T cell

Low	Small lymphocytic lymphoma
	Lymphoplasmacytic lymphoma/
	  Waldenstrom's
	  macroglobulinemia
	Marginal zone lymphomas
	Follicular lymphoma
	  (grades I and II)
		Sezary's syndrome/mycosis
		  fungoides
		Smoldering/chronic adult
		  T cell leukemia/
		  lymphoma

Intermediate	Mantle cell lymphoma Follicular lymphoma (grade III)	Peripheral T cell lymphoma Angioimmunoblastic lymphoma Angiocentric lymphoma Intestinal T cell lymphoma
High	Diffuse large B cell lymphoma Primary mediastinal B cell lymphoma Precursor B lymphoblastic Burkitt's lymphoma	Anaplastic large cell lymphoma Precursor T lymphoblastic Adult T cell leukemia/lymphoma

Fig. 16.1 The Revised American European Lymphoma (REAL) classification of non-Hodgkin's lymphoma.

Features of non-Hodgkin's lymphoma

- Superficial, asymmetric, painless lymphadenopathy
- Fever, night sweats, and weight loss
- Oropharyngeal involvement (5–10%)
- Cytopenias due to marrow failure or autoimmunity
- Abdominal disease (spleen, liver, MALT, and retroperitoneal/mesenteric nodes)

Fig. 16.2 Features of non-Hodgkin's lymphoma (MALT, mucosal-associated lymphoid tissue).

Clinical features of Hodgkin's disease

Painless, nontender lymphadenopathy: cervical then axillary nodes are most common, mediastinal in 10%
Splenomegaly (rarely massive)
Respiratory symptoms (mediastinal mass → superior vena cava obstruction)
Pruritus
Constitutional symptoms
- Weight loss
- Sweats
- High swinging "Pel-Ebstein" fever
- Alcohol-induced pain

Fig. 16.3 Clinical features of Hodgkin's disease.

Rye classification of Hodgkin's disease (HD)

Lymphocyte predominant	10% of cases of HD. The infiltrate consists of large numbers of lymphocytes and histiocytes, interspersed with a few RS cells. This subtype has a good prognosis
Nodular sclerosing	50% of cases of HD and, unlike other forms of HD, is more common in women. Broad bands of collagen fibers divide the lymph node into nodules containing a mixture of lymphocytes, eosinophils, plasma cells, macrophages, and lacunar cells
Mixed cellularity	30% of cases of HD. It is characterized by an infiltrate of histiocytes, plasma cells, and eosinophils. Fewer lymphocytes and more RS cells are present than in the lymphocyte-predominant form of the disease
Lymphocyte depletion	10% of cases of HD. RS cells or their variants are present in large numbers in conjunction with relatively few lymphocytes. Lymphocyte depletion has the poorest prognosis of all forms of HD

Fig. 16.4 Rye classification of Hodgkin's disease (HD) (RS, Reed-Sternberg).

Disease severity is directly proportional to the number of RS cells found in the lesions and indirectly linked to the number of lymphocytes in the lesions. RS cells are binucleated or multinucleated, with prominent eosinophilic nucleoli, giving an "owl's-eye" appearance. The clinical features of HD are shown in Fig. 16.3.

Hodgkin's disease has been classified into four histologic subtypes (Fig. 16.4). Although histologic composition is an important prognostic factor, clinical staging (Ann Arbor staging) is the most accurate indicator of long-term prognosis in HD (Fig. 16.5). Treatment depends on stage. Stages 1A and 2A receive radiotherapy, which cures 75–95%. Other stages receive combination chemotherapy over 6 months, but only 50–65% are cured. Late complications of the disease include the following:

- Infertility.
- Radiation pneumonitis.
- Pulmonary fibrosis.
- Secondary cancers, including AML.

Ann Arbor staging of malignant lymphomas	
Stage	Sites of involvement
I	Disease limited to single region of nodes or one extranodal site
II	Disease at two sites on the same side of the diaphragm
III	Disease at several sites on both sides of the diaphragm (includes spleen)
IV	Spread of disease to extra lymphatic structures (e.g., bone marrow, gut, lung, liver)

A: no symptoms
B: weight loss, sweats, fever

Fig. 16.5 Ann Arbor staging of malignant lymphomas.

Multiple myeloma

Multiple myeloma is a malignant proliferation of plasma cells in bone marrow, which produce a monoclonal paraprotein and/or light chain. The monoclonal immunoglobulin is found in serum, whereas the light-chain or Bence-Jones protein is found in urine. These monoclonal proteins form a discrete band on the electrophoretic strip (Fig. 16.6).

The incidence of multiple myeloma is 4–6 per 100,000 a year. It is a disease of late middle age and the elderly. Survival with adequate treatment (combination chemotherapy, thalidomide, localized radiotherapy) is 3–5 years. The etiology is unknown, apart from an increased incidence related to exposure to ionizing radiation. Tumor necrosis factor and interleukin-6 have been implicated in initiation of disease.

Diagnosis

Diagnosis requires the following:
- Monoclonal paraprotein in serum or urine.
- >10–15% plasma cells in the bone marrow.
- Osteolytic bone lesions on skeletal survey.

Clinical features

Bone destruction such as diffuse osteoporosis and pathologic fractures is a common feature. This is thought to arise as a result of bone resorption induced by the production of osteoclast-activating factor (OAF) by the myeloma cells. See Fig. 16.7 for the radiographic appearance of multiple myeloma.
- Neurologic symptoms are due to the compression of the spinal cord or roots by collapsed vertebrae.
- Normochromic normocytic anemia results from marrow infiltration.

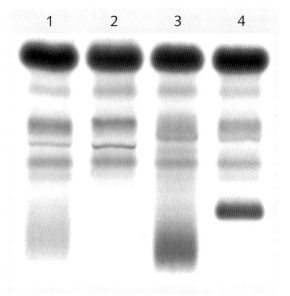

Fig. 16.6 Serum electrophoresis. Lane 1, normal sample; Lane 2, patient with antibody deficiency; Lane 3, patient with infection and polyclonal raised immunoglobulins; Lane 4, patient with myeloma and monoclonal immunoglobulins.

- Repeated infections can occur due to hypogammaglobulinemia and neutropenia.
- Hypercalcemia occurs in 10% of cases. This is due to increased reabsorption of bone and is indicative of advanced disease.
- Chronic renal failure occurs in 20–30% of patients. Factors that can contribute to renal failure in multiple myeloma are as follows:
  - Increased blood viscosity.
  - Hypercalcemia.
  - Renal tubular obstruction by proteinaceous casts.

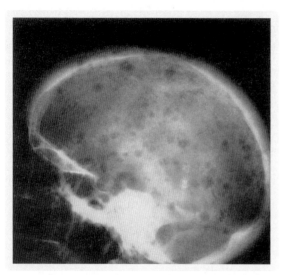

Fig. 16.7 Radiograph of the skull of a patient with multiple myeloma showing many osteolytic bone lesions (courtesy of Dr. M. Makris).

- ○ Toxic effect of Bence-Jones protein on proximal renal tubules.
- ○ Infection.
- ○ Dehydration.
- ○ Nonsteroidal anti-inflammatory drugs.
- ○ Light-chain deposition in glomeruli.
- Amyloidosis (see next column) can lead to nephrotic syndrome.
- An abnormal bleeding tendency occurs due to the adverse effect of paraprotein on platelets and coagulation factors.

Solitary myeloma (plasmacytoma)

A plasmacytoma is a solitary tumor found either in the bone or soft tissues, especially the upper respiratory tract. Osseous plasmacytomas usually progress to multiple myeloma. Extraosseous plasmacytomas do not disseminate, and, after excision and radiotherapy, prognosis is excellent.

Waldenström's macroglobulinemia

Waldenström's macroglobulinemia is a neoplastic monoclonal proliferation of cells derived from the B-cell lineage. A monoclonal IgM paraprotein (macroglobulin) is produced, increasing blood viscosity. Tumor cells are found in blood, bone marrow, lymph nodes, and spleen. The incidence is 3–6 per 100,000 a year and is higher in males than in females. Most patients present between the fifth and seventh decade. Survival averages 2–5 years. Bone pain and osteolytic lesions are rare, but hyperviscosity syndrome is common. Macroglobulin interferes with platelet function and coagulation factors, resulting in a tendency to bleed.

Heavy-chain disease

Heavy-chain disease is a rare condition in which tumor cells secrete incomplete immunoglobulin heavy chain. This is most commonly α heavy-chain disease (seen in Mediterranean countries). Heavy-chain disease can progress to lymphoma.

Monoclonal gammopathy of undetermined significance

Around 3% of people aged over 65 years have low levels of paraprotein without any symptom of disease. This condition is termed monoclonal gammopathy of uncertain significance (MGUS). There are <10% plasma cells in the marrow, no bone lesions, no anemia, and no renal failure; 10% will progress to myeloma within 10 years.

Amyloidosis

Amyloid is a heterogenous group of proteins that have a fibrillar ultrastructure, resulting in the formation of β-pleated sheets. Examples of amyloid proteins include:
- AA: serum amyloid A (SAA), an acute phase protein.
- AL: immunoglobulin light-chain or fragments.

In amyloidosis, amyloid is deposited in tissues. This can be localized or systemic, with renal impairment being a problem. Amyloidosis can occur in the following conditions:
- Chronic inflammatory disease (in which SAA is initially produced as an acute-phase response protein).
- Primary disease.
- Plasma cell disorders (multiple myeloma, Waldenström's macroglobulinemia).
- Long-term hemodialysis.

- Hereditary (very rare).
- Medullary carcinoma of the thyroid.
- Aging (cardiac or Alzheimer's disease).

Tumor immunology

The immune surveillance system prevents transformed cells from becoming tumors. In established tumors, several mechanisms allow this system to be eluded.

Investigations of tumor cells have demonstrated that many express antigens that are unique to the tumor. Such antigens include:
- Products of oncogenes or mutated tumor suppressor genes.
- A mutated or aberrantly expressed self-protein.
- An oncofetal antigen usually expressed only in early development.
- An oncogenic virus antigen.

These tumor-cell-associated antigens may be recognized by the immune system and lead to killing of the tumor cells by cytotoxic T cells, NK cells, macrophages, and antibodies. Fig. 16.8 demonstrates how the various parts of the immune system can respond to and destroy tumor cells.

The ability of the immune system to respond to and destroy tumor cells has been called the "immune surveillance system." Its efficacy is demonstrated practically by the fact that patients with primary and acquired immunodeficiencies and those on immunosuppressive therapy have a marked increase in the incidence of developing malignant tumors.

Tumor cells appear to evade the immune surveillance system by several mechanisms:
- As tumors develop and are attacked, selective outgrowth of antigen-negative cell variants arises.
- Tumor cells lose or decrease their expression of MHC molecules.
- Antigen masking.
- Expression of ligands that can lead to T-cell apoptosis.

The evasion of the immune surveillance system leads to growth of a clinically recognized tumor.

Use of immunology to manage tumors

Because tumor cells demonstrate unique antigens on their surface, monoclonal antibodies raised against these antibodies can be used for both diagnostic and therapeutic purposes. Efforts to stimulation cellular immune reactions against tumor cell antigens may also be useful in the treatment of tumors.

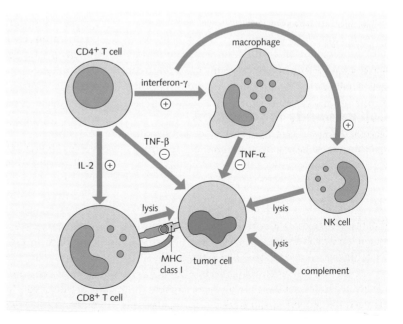

Fig. 16.8 The immune response to tumors. Both innate and adaptive immunity have been implicated in the response to tumors. Macrophages can inhibit tumor growth or cause cytotoxicity, probably through the release of tumor necrosis factor-alpha (TNF-α). Complement activation may also cause tumor cell lysis. Cytotoxic CD8$^+$ cells have been shown to lyse tumor cells *in vitro*. Many tumors evade T-cell cytotoxicity by reducing major histocompatibility complex (MHC) class I expression. This exposes them to lysis by natural killer (NK) cells. T helper cells activate cytotoxic T cells, macrophages, and NK cells. They also produce TNF-β, which inhibits tumor growth.

Neural antigens and associated paraneoplastic syndromes		
Antigen	**Syndrome**	**Associated tumor**
P-type VGCC	Myasthenic syndrome	Small cell lung cancer
Glutamate receptor	Cerebellar degeneration	Hodgkin's disease
HuD	Encephalomyelitis and sensory neuropathy	Small cell lung cancer Neuroblastoma
APCA-1	Cerebellar degeneration	Breast Ovary

Fig. 16.9 Neural antigens and associated paraneoplastic syndromes.

Antibodies in diagnosis

Injection of radio-labeled monoclonal antibodies directed against tumor antigens into an individual with that tumor followed by radioactivity body scanning can not only serve to delimit the extent of the main tumor but can also demonstrate sites of regional and distant spread. Several tumors also produce and secrete unique substances that can be detected in the serum by ELISA assays and can be used to monitor tumor burden.

Antibodies in treatment

Tumor-specific monoclonal antibodies can be injected into an individual with that tumor and lead to tumor cell killing on binding by the antibody engaging NK cells via its Fc receptor or by mediating complement activation and cytolysis. Currently, anti-CD20 is used in the treatment of B-cell lymphomas, and anti-Her-2 neu is used in treating breast and ovarian cancer patients whose tumors strongly express Her-2 neu. In development are antitumor monoclonal antibodies bound to toxins. These could result in specific delivery of the toxins by the antibodies to cause direct tumor cell killing.

Cell immunity in treatment

Several different approaches have been utilized in an attempt to use cell-mediated immunity in tumor treatment. Nonspecific activators of cellular immunity have been administered in an attempt to augment the immune surveillance system to control the tumor. Tumor cells have been modified *in vivo*, combined with adjuvants, and injected in hopes of stimulating a strong T-cell response. Tumor infiltrating lymphocytes (TILs) have been isolated from tumors, cloned *in vivo*, stimulated, and infused back into the patient, working on the assumption that these TILs represent T cells attempting to respond to the tumor.

Immunologically mediated paraneoplastic syndromes

The nervous system is an immunologically privileged site with many antigens not exposed to the systemic immune system because of the blood–brain barrier. If tumors outside the nervous system aberrantly express these antigens, an immune response can be mounted to these sequestered antigens. Paraneoplastic neurologic syndromes result from this immune response acting on the nervous system to cause neurologic degeneration or dysfunction. Paraneoplastic antineuronal antibodies are considered to be specific markers of malignancy.

Fig. 16.9 gives examples of neural antigens and associated paraneoplastic syndromes.

- What is leukemia?
- What are the clinical and laboratory findings in multiple myeloma?
- What is the difference between Hodgkin's and non-Hodgkin's lymphoma?
- What is amyloidosis?
- How does the immune system respond to tumors?
- What is a paraneoplastic syndrome?

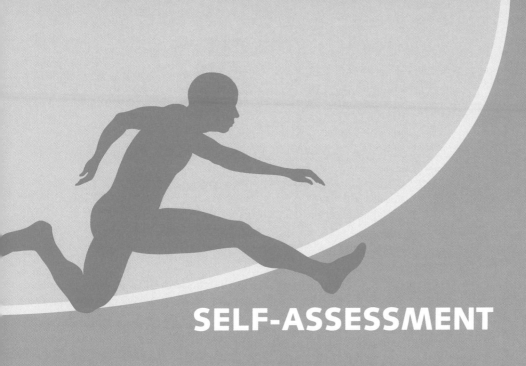

SELF-ASSESSMENT

Case Scenarios

Case 1

A 12-month-old boy is evaluated from recurrent serious bacterial infections. A complete blood count shows normal total numbers of neutrophils and lymphocysts. He has a lymphocyte profile by flow cytometry, which demonstrates normal CD3/CD4 and CD3/CD8 cells but no CD-19 cells. An immunoglobulin profile shows very low levels of IgM, IgG, and IgA.

1. What is his diagnosis?

(a) Chronic granulomatous disease.
(b) Agammaglobulinemia.
(c) Leukocyte adhesion defect.
(d) Hyper IgM syndrome.

2. His mother asks why he did not become ill sooner, because he has a primary immunodeficiency. You explain that:

(a) The condition is delayed because it is only after toxic intermediaries accumulate that immunocompetent cells are destroyed.
(b) Most pathogens cannot successfully attack small infants.
(c) Immunoglobulins transferred across the placenta provided passive protection early in life.

3. Your recommended therapy would be:

(a) Antibiotics on a daily basis.
(b) Immunoglobulin administration (IVIG).
(c) White cell transfusions.

Case 2

A 16-month-old boy has had recurrent bacterial infections, but they are not associated with pus formation. He has a consistently elevated neutrophil number in his blood. His immunoglobulin levels are normal.

1. What is his diagnosis?

(a) Chronic granulomatous disease.
(b) Leukocyte adhesion deficiency.
(c) Hyper-IgE syndrome.
(d) Agammaglobulinemia.

2. Laboratory testing diagnostic of his condition is:

(a) Absence of CD-11/CD-18 on the leukocyte membrane.
(b) Absence of selectins on the endothelial cell membranes.

(c) Failure of the neutrophils to produce a respiratory burst when activated.
(d) Inability to phagocytize encapsulated organisms.

Case 3

A 13-month-old boy develops recurrent serious bacterial infections. He has a complete blood count, which shows normal numbers of neutrophils and lymphocytes. An immunoglobulin profile shows high levels of IgM with absent IgG and IgA. A lymphocyte profile by flow cytometry shows normal numbers of CD3/CD4, CD3/CD8, and CD-19 positive cells. None of the child's lymphocytes express CD-154 (CD-40 ligand). A lymphocyte profile on his mother shows that only 40% of her lymphocytes express CD-154 (normal range 80–90%).

1. What is the diagnosis?

(a) Chronic granulomatous disease.
(b) Agammaglobulinemia.
(c) Severe combined immunodeficiency.
(d) Hyper-IgM syndrome.

2. His mother asks why she also has an abnormal flow cytometry result. You explain that the condition is:

(a) Autosomal dominant.
(b) Autosomal recessive.
(c) X-linked.

Case 4

A 4-year-old boy has recurrent respiratory and skin infections with *Staphylococcus aureus*. A perianal lesion is so severe and persistent that it is surgically removed. The pathologist calls to alert you that the central area shows granulomatous inflammation with neutrophils at the periphery.

1. What do you suspect that this patient's problem is?

(a) Leukocyte adhesion defect.
(b) Hyper-IgE syndrome.
(c) Selective IgA deficiency.
(d) Chronic granulomatous disease.

2. How would you prove your diagnosis?

(a) Demonstrate the failure of neutrophils to undergo a respiratory burst when stimulated.
(b) Show the absence of CD-11/CD-18 on neutrophils using flow cytometry.
(c) Measure the total hemolytic complement, and show it to be very low.
(d) Demonstrate the absence of serum IgG.

3. This condition is inherited as a/an:

(a) Autosomal recessive condition.
(b) Autosomal dominant condition.
(c) X-linked condition.
(d) A and B.
(e) A and C.

Case 5

A 27-year-old man presents with a diffuse pneumonia that is pathologically found to be due to *Pneumocystis* (PCP). Complete blood count shows a decrease in lymphocytes. The patient admits to intravenous drug abuse but has otherwise been healthy.

1. In view of the findings and history, the most important action would be to order:

(a) Immunoglobulin levels.
(b) Total hemolytic complement determination.
(c) Anti-HIV antibody.
(d) Lymphocyte mitogen stimulation.

2. A lymphocyte profile in this patient would probably demonstrate:

(a) Elevated CD-19 cells.
(b) Decreased CD3/CD8 cells.
(c) Decreased CD3/CD4 cells.
(d) Elevated CD-16 cells.

3. Based on the history, this patient is at increased risk for:

(a) Opportunistic infections.
(b) Neoplasia.
(c) Severe EBV infections.
(d) All of the above.

Case 6

A 43-year-old man is undergoing a second renal transplant. His previous transplant was lost to chronic rejection. Shortly after the establishment of blood flow during the transplant procedure, the donor kidney becomes swollen and hemorrhagic.

1. The likely cause of the kidney changes is:

(a) Hyperacute rejection.
(b) Ischemia.
(c) Acute cellular rejection.
(d) Chronic vascular rejection.

2. Appropriate therapy for this event is:

(a) Plasmapheresis.
(b) Steroid bolus.
(c) Administration of anti-CD3 antibody.
(d) Removal of the kidney.

Case 7

A 15-year-old girl presents with a "butterfly" rash on her cheeks, arthralgias, and blood in her urine. She demonstrates a positive antinuclear antigen and anti–double-stranded DNA in her serum. C3 levels are decreased.

1. The likely diagnosis is:

(a) Systemic lupus erythematosus.
(b) Bacterial sepsis.
(c) Graft versus host disease.
(d) Atopy.

2. A biopsy of the kidney would demonstrate:

(a) Granular immunofluorescent with anti-immunoglobulin and anti–C3-labeled antibodies.
(b) Glomerular electron dense deposits in EM examination.
(c) Glomerular capillary thrombi.
(d) Both A and B.

Case 8

A 5-year-old girl develops episodes of respiratory distress in the spring and has been hospitalized twice for treatment. Chest X-ray and tests for cystic fibrosis are negative. You suspect extrinsic asthma and perform skin testing with screening antigens. She develops a large area of skin edema and redness following a test for ragweed pollen.

1. What laboratory test would confirm your diagnosis of asthma due to ragweed pollen?

(a) High levels of anti-ragweed IgG in serum.
(b) High levels of anti-ragweed IgE in serum.
(c) High levels of anti-ragweed IgA in serum.
(d) High levels of anti-ragweed IgM in serum.

2. The girl will not take pills, and liquid medicines are a struggle for her mother to give. A good alternative approach might be:

(a) Periodic steroid injection.
(b) Desensitization (series of small dose antigen injection).
(c) Inhaled steroids.
(d) B and C.

Case 9

A 30-year-old woman with systemic lupus erythematosus (SLE) has undergone a renal transplant because of damage caused by her immune complex disease. She has received a kidney from a living, related donor who is a good (3/4 HLA sites match) match. The transplant went smoothly, and she is on a corticosteroid and cyclosporin. Ten months after transplant, she develops renal function problems. A kidney biopsy is performed and shows interstitial lymphocytic infiltrates and lymphocytes infiltrating tubules and destroying tubular cells.

Immunofluorescence shows no deposition of immunoglobulin or C3 in glomeruli.

1. Your diagnosis is:

(a) Recurrent lupus.
(b) Cyclosporin toxicity.
(c) Acute cellular rejection.
(d) Chronic vascular rejection.

2. The most appropriate acute therapy would be:

(a) Plasmapheresis to remove circulating immune complexes.
(b) Decrease in cyclosporin dosage.
(c) Administration of anti-CD3 antibody.
(d) Removal of the transplanted kidney.

Case 10

A 4-month-old girl presents with failure to grow normally. A complete blood count shows a decreased absolute number of lymphocytes. HIV serology is negative. A lymphocyte profile shows decreased CD3/CD4, CD3/CD8, and CD-19 cells. Immunoglobulin levels are low.

1. Your diagnosis is:

(a) Agammaglobulinemia.
(b) Chronic granulomatous disease.
(c) Severe combined immunodeficiency.
(d) Wiskott-Aldrich syndrome.

2. All of the following evaluations would be indicated except:

(a) Evaluation of lymphocyte blastogenic response to mitogens.
(b) Measurement of lymphocyte adenine deaminase levels.
(c) Evaluation for opportunistic pathogens such as *Candida* and *Pneumocystis*.
(d) Measurement of serum total hemolytic complement.

3. Definitive therapy for this condition would involve:

(a) Administration of steroids.
(b) Plasmapheresis.

(c) Granulocyte transfusions.
(d) Bone marrow transplantation.

Case 11

A 15-month-old child is brought to your office for well-child care. She requires her routine immunizations. She has a 5-year-old sibling who had a liver transplant 6 months ago and is still on high doses of corticosteroid.

1. Which immunization would you withhold because of her sibling's history?

(a) Hepatitis B.
(b) HIB (*Haemophilus influenzae*).
(c) Pneumococcal vaccine.
(d) MMR (measles, mumps, rubella).

2. The mother notes that the child has had mild upper respiratory symptoms but no fever. Is it still all right to immunize her?

(a) No.
(b) Yes.

Case 12

A 12-month-old child presents with eczema of the skin and thrombocytopenia and has had two serious bacterial infections. Complete blood count shows modest lymphopenia. Immunoglobulins are normal for the child's age.

1. Based on these findings the most likely diagnosis is:

(a) Chediak-Higashi syndrome.
(b) DiGeorge syndrome.
(c) Wiskott-Aldrich syndrome.
(d) Ataxia-telangiectasia syndrome.

2. A lymphocyte profile would likely demonstrate:

(a) Reduction of both CD3/CD4 and CD3/CD8 cells.
(b) Reduction of CD3/CD4 cells and elevation of CD3/CD8 cells.
(c) Normal CD3/CD4 and CD3/CD8 cells and decreased CD-19 cells.
(d) Only CD3/CD8 cells.

Case Scenario Answers

Case 1

The diagnosis is agammaglobulinemia. The history indicated no circulating B cells (no CD-19 positive cells) and virtually absent immunoglobulins. Onset of symptoms is delayed until the maternal immunoglobulins that were transmitted across the placental have been cleared (usually not before 3 months). This is likely Bruton agammaglobulinemia (X-linked form). Treatment is monthly intravenous immunoglobulin infusions. Chronic granulomatous disease and leukocyte adhesion defects are neutrophil disorders and would not be associated with absent B cells and very low immunoglobulins. Hyper-IgM syndrome is associated with normal B cell numbers and high IgM levels.
Answers: 1-b, 2-c, 3-b

Case 2

The diagnosis is leukocyte adhesion defect. The history indicates recurrent infections without pus formation, indicating a condition where neutrophils do not migrate to the site of infection. This could only result from an absence of neutrophils (he has an increased neutrophil count), an adhesion defect, or a defect in neutrophil chemotaxis (which is not given as an option). Chronic granulomatous disease is associated with abscess formation (due to failure of neutrophil oxidative killing), and agammaglobulinemia is a B-cell problem and does not affect neutrophils. Leukocyte adhesion is mediated through CD-11/-18, and its absence is the diagnostic test for this condition.
Answers: 1-b, 2-a

Case 3

The diagnosis is hyper-IgM syndrome. This is a condition caused by a failure of immunoglobulin class switching due to a lack of CD-154 (CD-40 ligand) on B cells. Normal numbers of B cells are present, and IgM is elevated with little IgG and IgA (ruling out a diagnosis of agammaglobulinemia). Normal T cell numbers are present, excluding a diagnosis of severe combined immunodeficiency. Chronic granulomatous disease would not be associated with

high IgM or the lack of CD-154 on B cells, as it is due to a neutrophil oxidative killing defect. Hyper-IgM syndrome is X-linked; flow cytometry studies would show the presence of CD-154 on half the mother's lymphocytes because of random X chromosome inactivation.
Answers: 1-d, 2-c

Case 4

The diagnosis is chronic granulomatous disease (CGD). The history of recurrent bacterial infections with catalase-producing organisms resulting in abscesses with granulomatous inflammation is characteristic. Leukocyte adhesion defect would not lead to granulomata. Hyper-IgE syndrome (Job syndrome) is not due to a failure of acute inflammation. Selective IgA deficiency is often asymptomatic and is not associated with granulomata formation. CGD is due to a failure of the generation of free radicals that result in oxidative killing (a failure of the "respiratory burst"). It is not associated with abnormalities in immunoglobulins or complement components. The oxidase, which is defective, results from the combination of a membrane bound and cytoplasmic component, one coded for on the X chromosome and one on autosomes, so CGD can be inherited as either an X-lined or autosomal recessive condition.
Answers: 1-d, 2-a, 3-d

Case 5

The diagnosis is HIV infection (AIDS). The history is one of an opportunistic infection associated with lymphocytopenia (due to decreased T helper cells) in an individual with risk-taking behavior (intravenous drug abuse). The appropriate first step in diagnosis is to look for evidence of antibodies to HIV; the other options do not apply to HIV infection until quite late in its course. As noted, the lymphocytes that are depleted are T helper cells (CD3/CD4 positive cells). HIV/AIDS is associated with a risk of opportunistic infection (in fact, this is one of the features that define AIDS), severe

EBV infections (as T cells important in control of EBV infection are depleted), and increased risk of neoplasia due to a failure of the "immune surveillance" system.
Answers: 1-c, 2-c, 3-d

Case 6

The diagnosis is hyperacute transplant rejection, which is a result of the presence of prefomed anti-HLA antibodies. The immediate time course and the fact that this is a second transplant make this diagnosis highly likely. The pathology is an acute vasculitis, which is associated with vascular damage, leading to a swollen and hemorrhagic kidney. There is no treatment for hyperacute rejection of the kidney except to remove the kidney.
Answers: 1-a, 2-d

Case 7

The diagnosis is systemic lupus erythematosus (SLE). "Butterfly" rash (photosensitivity), arthralgias, and glomerulonephritis (hematuria) are characteristic clinical findings of a systemic immune complex mediated disease. The positive antinuclear antibody (ANA) and especially anti-ds-DNA antibodies are characteristic of SLE. Low C3 levels are indicative of active disease, as they result from complement consumption. In an immune complex mediated disease, direct immunofluorescence of an affected tissue reveals granular deposition of immune complexes containing both immunoglobulin and complement. Electron microscopy of such a condition will reveal electron dense deposits, which are the actual immune complexes.
Answers: 1-a, 2-d

Case 8

The diagnosis in this case is an IgE-mediated immunopathologic process (atopy). Skin testing has demonstrated that an immediate hypersensitivity is evoked by ragweed pollen, so high levels of antiragweed IgE would be expected in the serum. IgE-mediated atopy can be treated by using mediator blockers (interfere with the initial phase), anti-inflammatory agents (interfere with the secondary phase associated with eosinophil accumulation), or by lowering levels of IgE through desensitization protocols. Systemic steroid therapy is used only in severe acute episodes; it is not used for preventive or chronic management because of its side effects.
Answers: 1-b, 2-d

Case 9

This is a case of an individual with SLE who underwent a living, related renal transplant because of SLE renal damage. It is now 10 months after the transplant, and the patient is having kidney problems and undergoes a renal biopsy. The major clinical concerns would be recurrent SLE in the transplant, some form of rejection, or cyclosporine toxicity (manifest as vascular damage and fibrosis). The absence of immune complexes in the biopsy excludes recurrent SLE. The tubulitis and interstitial lympocytic infiltrate are characteristic of acute cellular rejection. Acute cellular rejection is the only form of rejection for which there is reasonable treatment. Use of anti-CD3 antibodies to destroy the infiltrating lymphocytes is the correct approach. Plasmapheresis would not be of value, as the rejection is cell mediated. Decreasing the cyclosporine would make matters worse.
Answers: 1-c, 2-c

Case 10

This is a case of primary severe combined immunodeficiency (SCID). Both T cells and B cells are decreased, and there is no evidence of HIV infection, which would be the acquired cause to consider. You would be concerned about possible opportunistic infections and want to evaluate residual lymphocyte function and try to find the underlying cause (ADA measurements), but it is unlikely complement function is altered. Cellular immunodeficiencies are treated by stem-cell transplants.
Answers: 1-c, 2-d, 3-d

Case 11

This is a case of a normal child with an immunocompromised sibling. You would not want to administer a live viral vaccine to this child because of the potential to infect the immunocompromised sibling. Mild respiratory illnesses are not a reason to withhold immunizations.
Answers: 1-d, 2-b

Case 12

This child has Wiskott-Aldrich syndrome.
You are given a choice of the four major primary immunodeficiency syndromes that have characteristic physical findings: Chediak-Higashi (albinism, abnormal granules in leukocytes), DiGeorge (facial dysmorphism, absent thymus, absent parathyroids, and cardiac disease), ataxia-telangiectasia (abnormal gait and telangiectasia), and Wiskott-Aldrich (eczema and thrombocytopenia). In this syndrome, the numbers of both T helper and suppressor cells are decreased.

Answers: 1-c, 2-a

Multiple-Choice Questions

Indicate whether each answer is true or false

1. **Which of the following characteristics of tumor cells can activate an immune response:**

   (a) Viral antigens.
   (b) Embryonic antigens.
   (c) Glycosylated variants of normal self-proteins.
   (d) Absence of MHC class I molecules.
   (e) High concentrations of normal self-proteins.

2. **Regarding the immune system:**

   (a) An antigen is a molecule that can be recognized by the adaptive immune system.
   (b) Antibody isotypes are antibodies that bind to other antibodies.
   (c) Haptens are not immunogenic by themselves.
   (d) Lymph nodes are primary lymphoid organs.
   (e) The innate immune system exhibits immunological memory.

3. **In comparison to monocytes, macrophages:**

   (a) Are smaller.
   (b) Live longer.
   (c) Have greater phagocytic ability.
   (d) Are more likely to be found in the circulation.
   (e) Produce more lytic enzymes.

4. **Macrophages can be activated by:**

   (a) Interferon-γ.
   (b) Complement.
   (c) Coagulation products.
   (d) Interleukin-2.
   (e) Fas ligand.

5. **In comparison to macrophages, neutrophils:**

   (a) Are longer lived.
   (b) Can control mycobacteria.
   (c) Communicate with T cells.
   (d) Can present exogenous antigen.
   (e) Move and phagocytose more quickly.

6. **Which of the following are products of oxygen-dependent pathways:**

   (a) Superoxide radicals.
   (b) Hypochlorus acid.
   (c) Lysozyme.
   (d) Hydrogen peroxide.
   (e) Cationic proteins.

7. **Concerning natural killer cells:**

   (a) They are activated by specific, individual antigens.
   (b) They can detect classical and nonclassical MHC class I molecules.
   (c) They are involved in antibody-dependent cell-mediated cytotoxicity.
   (d) Because they are lymphoid cells, they exhibit immunologic memory.
   (e) They cause cellular necrosis.

8. **Concerning the complement system:**

   (a) The classical pathway is activated by MHC molecules.
   (b) It can be activated by bacterial carbohydrates.
   (c) It can activate spontaneously.
   (d) It causes ion-permeable pores to form in target cells.
   (e) It is involved in the recruitment of inflammatory cells.

9. **Which of the following inhibitors of complement are linked with the correct actions:**

   (a) Factor H inactivates C5 convertase.
   (b) Decay accelerating factor speeds up the decay of the membrane attack complex.
   (c) Factor I cleaves C3b and C4b.
   (d) CD-59 prevents the membrane attack complex from forming.
   (e) C1 inhibitor inhibits C1.

10. **Which of the following are members of the immunoglobulin gene superfamily:**

    (a) T cell receptor.
    (b) CD3-ζ.
    (c) Human leukocyte antigen molecules.
    (d) ICAM-1.
    (e) Polyimmunoglobulin receptor.

11. **Concerning primary and secondary lymphoid tissue:**

    (a) The thymus is a secondary lymphoid organ.
    (b) Lymph node germinal follicles contain mainly T cells.

(c) B-cell hypermutation occurs in the bone marrow.
(d) Lymph nodes sample antigen from the blood.
(e) Peyer's patches are part of the mucosal-associated lymphoid tissue.

12. Concerning generation of antigen receptor diversity:

(a) Both the light and heavy immunoglobulin chain variable regions are encoded by V, D, and J gene segments.
(b) Diversity can only be generated before encountering antigen.
(c) Somatic hypermutation occurs in both B and T cells.
(d) Antibodies produced late in an immune response have increased affinity for antigen.
(e) Each person's T-cell receptor repertoire will be the same.

13. IgA:

(a) Is important in mucosal immunity.
(b) Is found in breast milk.
(c) Is the most abundant immunoglobulin in the blood.
(d) Crosses the placenta.
(e) Is normally a dimer.

14. The major histocompatibility complex (MHC):

(a) Encodes human leukocyte antigen (HLA) molecules.
(b) Is located on chromosome 16 in humans.
(c) Encodes some complement components.
(d) Contains the gene for TNF.
(e) Encodes β_2-microglobulin.

15. Concerning the acute phase response:

(a) There is a change in the concentration of a number of plasma proteins.
(b) Leukocytosis and thrombocytopenia develop.
(c) Levels of ceruloplasmin and α_1-glycoprotein undergo a 100- to 1000-fold increase.
(d) Levels of C-reactive protein and serum amyloid A rise within hours of tissue injury.
(e) There is a decrease in plasma viscosity.

16. Concerning class I MHC molecules:

(a) A class I molecule is made up of α- and β-chains.
(b) CD8$^+$ T cells are class I MHC-restricted.
(c) Class I molecules are present only on antigen-presenting cells.
(d) Class I molecules present endogenous antigen.
(e) A class I molecule can bind longer peptides than a class II molecule because the peptide-binding cleft is more open.

17. Concerning recognition molecules of the immune system:

(a) Immunoglobulin molecules consist of two heavy chains and two light chains.
(b) The variable regions of the heavy and light chains are identical.
(c) The framework regions of immunoglobulins comprise the antigen-binding site.
(d) TCR signals are transduced by Igα/Igβ.
(e) Approximately 95% of T cells express $\gamma\delta$ receptors.

18. The following are components of the innate immune system:

(a) Interferons α and β.
(b) T cells.
(c) Complement.
(d) Antibody.
(e) Acute-phase proteins.

19. DiGeorge syndrome is characterized by:

(a) Malformation of the third and fourth pharyngeal pouches.
(b) Thymic hyperplasia.
(c) Hyperparathyroidism.
(d) Cardiac defects.
(e) Recurrent infections.

20. Regarding the complement system:

(a) Complement components are proteins or glycoproteins.
(b) Complement can only be activated by the alternative and classical pathways.
(c) The alternative pathway is usually activated by IgM and IgG.
(d) Complement components C5, C6, C7, C8, and C9 comprise the membrane attack complex.
(e) The conversion of C3 to C3b by C3 convertase is the major amplification process in the complement cascade.

21. Concerning lymph nodes:

(a) Antigen enters lymph nodes from the blood.
(b) Lymph filters from the cortex to the medulla.
(c) They contain B cells, T cells, and antigen-presenting cells.
(d) Lymphocytes can enter the node directly from the blood.
(e) They act to pump lymph around the body.

22. The following are examples of mucosal-associated lymphoid tissue (MALT):

(a) Tonsils.
(b) Appendix.

(c) Thymus.
(d) Peyer's patches.
(e) Inguinal lymph nodes.

23. The thymus:

(a) Is a bilobed gland.
(b) Is usually located in the neck.
(c) Exhibits a high rate of cell death.
(d) Contains stromal cells that support developing neutrophils.
(e) Produces hormones that control T cell maturation.

24. T helper cells:

(a) Express CD4.
(b) Are required for antibody production against protein antigens.
(c) Produce a wide variety of cytokines, which stimulate the innate and adaptive immune systems.
(d) Do not express T-cell receptors.
(e) Determine the type of adaptive immune response mounted.

25. Concerning acute inflammation:

(a) Acute inflammation is characterized by infiltration of neutrophils and vascular changes.
(b) TNF-α is an important mediator.
(c) The complement system does not play a role.
(d) The coagulation and fibrinolytic systems are activated.
(e) ICAM-1 and ICAM-2 are downregulated.

26. The actions of cytokines in acute inflammation include:

(a) Induction of adhesion molecules.
(b) Induction of cell membrane phospholipid and prostaglandin metabolism.
(c) Chemotaxis of neutrophils.
(d) Stimulate fibroblast proliferation.
(e) Mediate the acute phase response.

27. Which of the following are arachidonic acid metabolites:

(a) Platelet-activating factor.
(b) Leukotriene B_4.
(c) Thromboxane A_2.
(d) Perforin.
(e) Prostacyclin.

28. Concerning leukocyte margination, and extravasation in acute inflammation:

(a) Neutrophils are important in the early part of the response.

(b) Selectin molecules expressed constitutively on endothelial cells bind to selectin molecules on leukocytes.
(c) The interaction between leukocytes and endothelium is strengthened by integrin molecules.
(d) Integrin molecules are important for leukocyte homing.
(e) The endothelial cells form pores large enough for spherical leukocytes to pass through.

29. Concerning chronic inflammation:

(a) Neutrophils form the majority of cells present.
(b) The macrophage plays a central role.
(c) Granuloma formation is a characteristic feature.
(d) TNF-α is crucial in granuloma maintenance.
(e) Lymphocytes are not usually present.

30. The following are potential consequences of chronic inflammation:

(a) Tissue injury.
(b) The tissue returns to normal.
(c) Weight loss and fever.
(d) Adaptive immune system activation.
(e) Fibrosis.

31. Which of the following are important for the immune response to viruses:

(a) Lysozyme.
(b) Antibody.
(c) Interferons.
(d) Eosinophils.
(e) Cytotoxic T cells.

32. Viruses evade the normal immune response by:

(a) Undergoing mutation between epidemics.
(b) Reducing MHC class I expression.
(c) Mutating within the host.
(d) Releasing exotoxins.
(e) Becoming latent.

33. Protozoal infection is often chronic because:

(a) They have marked antigenic variation.
(b) They are immunosuppressive.
(c) They have complex lifecycles.
(d) Infection is intracellular.
(e) They can escape into the cytoplasm following phagocytosis.

34. Regarding hypersensitivity reactions:

(a) Type I hypersensitivity reactions are mediated by IgG.

(b) Type III hypersensitivity involves the formation of immune complexes.
(c) Mast cells play a key role in immediate hypersensitivity.
(d) Delayed-type hypersensitivity mechanisms play a key role in hemolytic disease of the newborn due to rhesus incompatibility.
(e) The Arthus reaction is a localized type III reaction.

35. The following are examples of hypersensitivity reactions:

(a) A positive skin-prick test.
(b) A positive Mantoux or PPD test.
(c) Hay fever.
(d) Graves' disease.
(e) Osteoarthritis.

36. Concerning anti-inflammatory drugs:

(a) Acetaminophen is an excellent anti-inflammatory.
(b) Steroids can only be given intravenously.
(c) NSAIDs act by inhibiting phospholipase A_2.
(d) Anti-TNF-α is anti-inflammatory.
(e) NSAIDs may be nephrotoxic and cause bronchospasm.

37. Concerning allergies:

(a) They are always type I hypersensitivity reactions.
(b) Asthma is characterized by reversible airway obstruction.
(c) Pollen and dust-mite feces are common allergens.
(d) Atopy refers to a predisposition to allergic conditions.
(e) Anaphylaxis is associated with hypertension.

38. Concerning treatment of allergies:

(a) Controlled exposure to low doses of antigen can be helpful.
(b) Antihistamines cure many allergic conditions.
(c) Steroids are useful.
(d) Epineprhine is commonly needed in the treatment of severe anaphylaxis.
(e) Prophylactic treatment often reduces the occurrence of symptoms.

39. Self-tolerance can be due to:

(a) Early clonal deletion.
(b) Clonal anergy.
(c) Molecular mimicry.
(d) Fas ligand expression.
(e) Regulatory T cells.

40. Concerning systemic lupus erythematosus (SLE):

(a) SLE is an organ-specific autoimmune disease.
(b) SLE is more common in men than women.
(c) SLE is characterized by antinuclear autoantibodies.
(d) The presence of HLA-DR5 and HLA-DR6 haplotypes confers an increased risk of developing SLE.
(e) An erythematous rash is common.

41. Concerning rheumatoid arthritis (RA):

(a) RA is characterized by inflammation of the synovium and destruction of the articular cartilage.
(b) Inflammation is limited to joints.
(c) TNF is a key cytokine in pathogenesis.
(d) RA is more common in women than in men.
(e) Type II collagen is the major autoantigen.

42. Rheumatoid factor:

(a) Is found in all cases of rheumatoid arthritis.
(b) Is an autoantibody.
(c) Is directed against IgM.
(d) Can activate complement.
(e) Amplifies the inflammatory response.

43. The following autoimmune diseases are organ specific:

(a) Reiter's syndrome.
(b) Hashimoto's thyroiditis.
(c) Myasthenia gravis.
(d) Graves' disease.
(e) Polyarteritis nodosa.

44. The following are examples of primary immunodeficiencies:

(a) Chronic granulomatous disease.
(b) Transient hypogammaglobulinemia of infancy.
(c) Splenectomy.
(d) AIDS.
(e) Wiskott-Aldrich syndrome.

45. Antibody deficiency can present with:

(a) Bronchiectasis.
(b) Diarrhea.
(c) Rheumatoid arthritis.
(d) Hyperviscosity.
(e) Mycoplasma joint infections.

46. Features of HIV include:

(a) Polyclonal B-cell activation.
(b) Defective T-cell function.

(c) Low rate of viral replication during asymptomatic phase.
(d) Antibodies directed against gp120 and gp41.
(e) Persistent generalized lymphadenopathy.

47. During HIV infection, which of the following infections are common:

(a) CMV retinitis.
(b) *Pneumocystis carinii.*
(c) Esophageal candidiasis.
(d) *Mycobacterium avium intracellulare* (MAC).
(e) Toxoplasmosis.

48. Concerning the routine immunization schedule in the U.S.:

(a) MMR is given at 2, 3, and 4 months.
(b) BCG is given neonatally or at 10–14 years.
(c) Influenza vaccine is given to people over 65 years of age.
(d) Tetanus vaccine requires boosters.

49. Live vaccines are used to prevent:

(a) Polio.
(b) Tetanus.
(c) Rubella.
(d) Hepatitis B.

50. Concerning mechanisms of transplant rejection:

(a) Hyperacute rejection only occurs once the recipient has synthesized antibody to the graft.
(b) Acute cellular rejection is primarily mediated by natural killer cells.
(c) Acute rejection is due to antidonor antibodies.
(d) Chronic rejection may be due to several mechanisms.
(e) Complement is implicated in hyperacute rejection.

51. The risk of transplant rejection can be reduced by:

(a) Using a graft from a monozygous twin.
(b) Using steroids.
(c) Using monoclonal antibodies.
(d) Using unmatched grafts.

52. Bone marrow:

(a) Is the main site of hematopoiesis in adults.
(b) Is found throughout the skeleton of newborns.
(c) Contains a large amount of fat.
(d) Contains macrophages important for the transfer of iron to developing erythrocytes.
(e) Forms T-lymphocyte precursors.

53. Regarding the spleen:

(a) The spleen is normally anterior to the stomach.
(b) The red pulp removes old or defective erythrocytes from the circulation.
(c) There are usually more primary than secondary B-cell follicles.
(d) Develops from the primitive gut.
(e) Primary cancers are rare.

54. Hematopoietic stem cells:

(a) Are found only in the bone marrow.
(b) Are able to produce plasma cells.
(c) Can self-replicate.
(d) Become lineage-committed precursor cells.
(e) Need growth factors to differentiate.

55. Polymorphonuclear leukocytes:

(a) Have a large round nucleus.
(b) Primarily respond to parasitic infections.
(c) Are granulocytes.
(d) Are phagocytic.
(e) Are a major constituent of pus.

56. Which of the following are consistent with a diagnosis of non-Hodgkin's lymphoma:

(a) Painless lymphadenopathy.
(b) Reed-Sternberg cells in the lesion.
(c) Fever, night sweats, and weight loss.
(d) Fanconi's syndrome.
(e) HIV infection.

57. A macrophage:

(a) Is a differentiated monocyte.
(b) Is capable of phagocytosis.
(c) May play an important role in the adaptive immune response.
(d) Can be infected by HIV.
(e) Is central to the allergic response.

58. Chronic lymphocytic leukemia:

(a) Is the most common leukemia.
(b) Is rapidly progressive.
(c) Is usually of B-cell origin.
(d) Is commonly associated with autoimmune hemolytic anemia.
(e) Converts to acute leukemia within 5 years.

59. Regarding acute lymphoblastic leukemia:

(a) It is the most common leukemia in children.
(b) Presentation after 10 years of age is associated with a poorer prognosis.

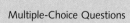

(c) Remission rates are low.
(d) It is commonly of T-cell origin.
(e) It may be caused by radiation exposure.

60. Acute myeloblastic leukemia:

(a) Is caused by an accumulation of differentiated myeloid cells in the bone marrow.
(b) Is associated with Down syndrome.
(c) Is characterized by isochromosome 12p.
(d) Has a better prognosis in older patients.
(e) May present with bleeding.

61. Regarding chronic myeloid leukemia:

(a) It is often identified in chronic phase.
(b) <10% of patients develop to an accelerated phase within 10 years of diagnosis.
(c) The Philadelphia chromosome is a disease marker.
(d) Treatment may be with Glivec.
(e) Bone marrow transplant is potentially curative.

62. Which of the following are features of multiple myeloma:

(a) Bence-Jones protein in the plasma.
(b) Presentation with paraplegia.
(c) Repeated infections.
(d) Bone destruction.
(e) >10% plasma cells in the marrow.

63. Regarding the ABO antigen system:

(a) People who are blood group O must have two parents who are both blood group O.
(b) People who are blood group A will produce anti-B antibodies.
(c) In group O, the T antigen is left unchanged.
(d) Group AB people will usually produce a hemolytic reaction to group O blood.
(e) Anti-A and anti-B antibodies are usually IgG.

64. Hemolytic disease of the newborn:

(a) Is commonly due to rhesus D incompatibility.
(b) Usually occurs in the first child.
(c) Will not occur if the mother is rhesus D positive.
(d) Can be prevented by passive immunization.
(e) Is due to IgM antibodies.

65. Regarding acute hemolytic transfusion reactions:

(a) They are caused by the destruction of donor red blood cells by antibodies present in the recipient's serum.
(b) They may lead to complement activation.
(c) They develop a few days after transfusion.
(d) Hypertension, flushing, urticaria, diarrhea, and vomiting ensue.
(e) They may cause disseminated intravascular coagulation.

1. (a) T—Tumors induced by viral infection can express viral antigens.
   (b) T—Carcinoembryonic antigen is seen in colonic cancer; α-fetoprotein in liver cancers.
   (c) T—Normal cell proteins can become abnormally glycosylated in tumors.
   (d) T—Absence of MHC class I can stimulate NK cells.
   (e) F—Completely normal proteins cannot stimulate the immune system.

2. (a) T—Antigens are recognized by the adaptive immune system.
   (b) F—Isotypes are different classes of antibody.
   (c) T—Haptens require large carrier molecules to elicit an immune response.
   (d) F—Lymph nodes are secondary lymphoid organs.
   (e) F—The innate immune system does not exhibit memory.

3. (a) F—Macrophages are larger than monocytes.
   (b) T—Macrophages can survive for many years within the tissues.
   (c) T—Macrophages are primarily phagocytic.
   (d) F—Macrophages form from monocytes when they enter tissues.
   (e) T—Lytic enzymes are produced to improve destruction of phagocytosed material.

4. (a) T—Cytokines, including IFN-γ, activate macrophages.
   (b) T—Complement acts as an opsonin for phagocytes.
   (c) T—Coagulation products activate macrophages.
   (d) F—IL-2 is a T-cell growth factor.
   (e) F—Fas ligand will cause cells expressing Fas to undergo apoptosis.

5. (a) F—Macrophages are longer lived; neutrophils die soon after dealing with pathogens.
   (b) F—Macrophages are required to control mycobacteria.
   (c) F—Macrophages, but not neutrophils, stimulate T cells by secreting IL-12.
   (d) F—Neutrophils do not process exogenous antigen or produce MHC class II to present antigen.
   (e) T—Neutrophils move and phagocytose more quickly than macrophages.

6. (a) T—Superoxide radicals are produced from molecular oxygen.
   (b) T—Hypochlorus acid is produced when myeloperoxidase catalyses a reaction between hydrogen peroxide and chloride ions.
   (c) F—Lysozyme is oxygen independent and acts to split peptidoglycan.
   (d) T—Hydrogen peroxide is formed when superoxide radicals combine with hydrogen ions.
   (e) F—Cationic proteins are oxygen independent and damage microbial membranes.

7. (a) F—Natural killer cells do not recognize specific individual antigens, but characteristics of cells such as the level of MHC expression.
   (b) T—KIRs detect classical MHC class I; CD94: NKG2 detects nonclassical MHC class I.
   (c) T—Natural killer cells can kill antibody-coated cells irrespective of the presence of MHC.
   (d) F—Natural killer cells are part of the innate immune system and do not exhibit memory.
   (e) F—Killing is via apoptosis.

8. (a) F—The classical pathway is activated by antibody bound to antigen.
   (b) T—The lectin pathway is activated when mannan-binding lectin binds to bacterial carbohydrates.
   (c) T—The alternative pathway starts with spontaneous activation of C3.
   (d) T—Complement killing is by formation of the membrane attack complex.
   (e) T—Complement recruits inflammatory cells and kills or opsonizes pathogens.

9. (a) F—Factor H prevents assembly of C3 convertase.
   (b) F—Decay accelerating factor accelerates the decay of C3 convertase.
   (c) T—Factor I and membrane cofactor protein cleave C3b and C4b.
   (d) T—CD59 (protectin) prevents the membrane attack complex from forming.
   (e) T—C1 inhibitor inhibits C1.

10. (a) T—The T cell receptor consists of four immunoglobulin domains.
    (b) F—CD3-ε, -γ, and -δ contain immunoglobulin domains, but ζ does not.
    (c) T—HLA molecules consist of four immunoglobulin domains.
    (d) T—Certain adhesion molecules, including ICAM-1, are members of the immunoglobulin gene superfamily.
    (e) T—The polyimmunoglobulin receptor is a member of the immunoglobulin gene superfamily.

11. (a) F—T cell maturation occurs in the thymus; therefore, it is a primary lymphoid organ.

(b) F—Lymph node germinal follicles are primarily composed of B cells.

(c) F—Diversity in immunoglobulin molecules is generated in the bone marrow, but somatic hypermutation occurs within germinal centers.

(d) F—Lymph nodes sample antigen from lymph (fluid drained from interstitial tissues).

(e) T—Peyer's patches are organized mucosal-associated lymphoid organs.

12. (a) F—The light chain has only V and J segments.

(b) F—Somatic hypermutation of immunoglobulin occurs after encountering antigen.

(c) F—T cells do not undergo somatic hypermutation.

(d) T—Antibody affinity increases during an immune response because of somatic hypermutation.

(e) F—The T-cell receptor repertoire depends on HLA molecules, which are polymorphic.

13. (a) T—IgA is secreted across mucosal surfaces.

(b) T—IgA is also secreted in breast milk.

(c) F—IgG is the most abundant immunoglobulin in blood.

(d) F—IgG, not IgA, crosses the placenta.

(e) T—IgA is usually dimeric.

14. (a) T—HLA molecules are human MHC molecules.

(b) F—The HLA complex is found on chromosome 6.

(c) T—The class III region of HLA encodes C4 and C2.

(d) T—The TNF gene is encoded within the MHC.

(e) F—β_2-microglobulin is not encoded on chromosome 6.

15. (a) T—The acute phase plasma proteins increase in concentration.

(b) F—Thrombocytosis develops.

(c) F—Levels of ceruloplasmin rise to about 150% of normal levels.

(d) T—CRP and SAA rise rapidly.

(e) F—Plasma viscosity and ESR are raised.

16. (a) F—Class I molecules are formed from α-chains and β_2-microglobulin.

(b) T—CD8$^+$ T cells are class I MHC-restricted, targeting them to endogenous antigen presentation.

(c) F—All nucleated cells express class I molecules.

(d) T—Class I molecules present endogenous antigen.

(e) F—Class I molecules present peptides 9 amino acids long, class II present peptides 12–15 peptides long.

17. (a) T—Each immunoglobulin molecule consists of two identical heavy chains and two identical light chains.

(b) F—The variable regions of the heavy and light chains are derived from different genetic recombination events.

(c) F—The variable regions comprise the antigen-binding site.

(d) F—TCR signals through CD3.

(e) F—Approximately 5% of T cells express $\alpha\beta$ receptors.

18. (a) T—Interferons α and β are produced by a wide number of cells to induce an antiviral state (γ-interferon is produced by T cells).

(b) F—T cells are part of the adaptive immune response.

(c) T—The complement system is a cascade of proteins involved in the innate immune system.

(d) F—Antibodies are specific and therefore part of the adaptive response.

(e) T—Acute-phase proteins are innate molecules.

19. (a) T—Malformation of the third and fourth pharyngeal pouches can lead to failure of thymic development.

(b) F—In DiGeorge syndrome, the thymus is hypoplastic.

(c) F—The parathyroid glands also fail to develop.

(d) T—Cardiac defects occurs in DiGeorge syndrome.

(e) T—Recurrent infections occur in DiGeorge syndrome because of the lack of T cells.

20. (a) T—Complement proteins are proenzymes.

(b) F—Complement can also be activated by lectins, which bind bacteria.

(c) F—The alternative pathway is activated spontaneously, particularly on cell surfaces.

(d) T—The MAC is formed from C5, C6, C7, C8, and C9.

(e) T—C3 convertase provides a major amplification step.

21. (a) F—Antigen enters lymph nodes via lymphatics.

(b) T—Lymph filters from the outside to the inside of the node.

(c) T—Lymph nodes provide an environment for T- and B-cell activation.

(d) T—Lymphocytes leave the blood through high endothelial vessels.

(e) F—Lymph circulates passively.

22. (a) T—Pharyngeal tonsils are organized MALT.

(b) T—The appendix is an organized MALT found in the cecum.

(c) F—The thymus is a secondary lymphoid organ not associated with the mucosa.

(d) T—Peyer's patches are organized MALT found throughout the small and large intestine.

(e) F—Inguinal lymph nodes drain lymph from the lower limbs.

23. (a) T—The thymus is bilobed.

(b) F—The thymus is normally found in the mediastinum, but can extend into the neck.

(c) T—Over 95% of T-cell precursors undergo apoptosis in the thymus.

(d) F—Stromal cells support developing thymocytes.

(e) T—Thymic epithelial cells produce several hormones that are essential for the differentiation and maturation of thymocytes.

24. (a) T—T helper cells are usually CD4$^+$.
   (b) T—T-cell help is required to produce antibodies against protein antigens.
   (c) T—Cytokines produced by T cells are important in the adaptive and innate immune responses.
   (d) F—T helper cells express TCRs in order to detect MHC class II molecules and antigen on APCs.
   (e) T—Different T helper subsets mediate antibody or cell-mediated responses.

25. (a) T—Vascular changes and neutrophil infiltration are mediated by several chemical mediators.
   (b) T—TNF-α is one of the important mediators.
   (c) F—Activation of the complement system produces important mediators for acute inflammation.
   (d) T—Coagulation and fibrinolytic systems are also involved in acute inflammation.
   (e) F—ICAM molecules are upregulated on endothelial cells.

26. (a) T—Adhesion molecules are induced on the endothelium.
   (b) T—Production of platelet-activating factor and prostacyclin is increased.
   (c) T—Neutrophils are attracted by chemotactic cytokines.
   (d) T—Fibroblasts proliferate and increase collagen synthesis.
   (e) T—Cytokines are involved in the development of the acute phase response.

27. (a) F—PAF is produced from cell membrane phospholipids but not from arachidonic acid.
   (b) T—Leukotriene B$_4$ is produced from 5-HPETE, a metabolite of arachidonic acid.
   (c) T—Thromboxane A$_2$ is an endoperoxide produced from the metabolism of arachidonic acid.
   (d) F—Perforin is produced and stored in vesicles in cytotoxic T cells and natural killer cells.
   (e) T—Prostacyclin is an endoperoxide produced from the metabolism of arachidonic acid.

28. (a) T—Neutrophils are the first cells to sites of inflammation.
   (b) F—L-selectin is constitutively expressed by leukocytes, whereas E- and P-selectin must be induced on endothelial cells.
   (c) T—Integrin molecules are rapidly induced and strengthen binding.
   (d) T—Integrin molecules such as $\alpha_4\beta_7$ are important for leukocyte homing.
   (e) F—Leukocytes change shape to move between endothelial cells.

29. (a) F—Macrophages, and not neutrophils, dominate chronic inflammation.
   (b) T—Macrophages are central to chronic inflammation.
   (c) T—Granulomas can result as part of a chronic inflammatory process.
   (d) T—TNF-α is needed for granuloma formation and maintenance.
   (e) F—Lymphocytes are always involved in chronic inflammatory responses.

30. (a) T—Tissue injury is caused by release of several mediators, including toxic oxygen metabolites.
   (b) F—A chronic inflammatory response will persist or result in scar formation.
   (c) T—Systemic features, such as weight loss and persistent fever, are characteristic features of chronic inflammation.
   (d) T—Macrophages present antigen to T cells.
   (e) T—Macrophages release fibrogenic cytokines.

31. (a) F—Lysozyme is an important part of the innate response to bacteria.
   (b) T—Antibodies can bind to free virus, preventing entry to cells and increasing phagocytosis.
   (c) T—Interferons induce antiviral states in uninfected cells and activate.
   (d) F—Eosinophils are involved in the response against large extracellular parasites such as helminths.
   (e) T—Cytotoxic T cells recognize virally infected cells and kill them.

32. (a) T—Some viruses undergo gradual mutation; the new mutant strain causes a fresh epidemic every few years (e.g., influenza).
   (b) T—MHC expression is reduced by several viruses, including CMV, EBV, and adenovirus.
   (c) T—Viruses with unstable genomes (e.g., HIV) undergo mutation within the host. The mutated viruses escape the immune system.
   (d) F—Some bacteria release exotoxins. Viral genomes are too small to encode exotoxins.
   (e) T—HSV, EBV, and varicella-zoster can become latent.

33. (a) T—Antigenic variation circumvents immunological memory.
   (b) T—Trypanosomes and malaria are immunosuppressive.
   (c) T—Protozoa often have several different stages during infection, thereby presenting several challenges to the immune system.
   (d) T—By infecting intracellularly, humoral immunity is less effective.
   (e) T—Trypanosomes can escape from phagosomes into the cytoplasm.

34. (a) F—IgE mediates type I reactions.
   (b) T—Complexes composed of antigen and antibody cause type III hypersensitivity.

119

(c) T—Mast-cell degranulation causes type I hypersensitivity.

(d) F—Rhesus incompatibility is a type II hypersensitivity reaction.

(e) T—In the Arthus reaction, immune complexes are deposited in the tissues.

35. (a) T—The skin-prick test is for type I (allergic) hypersensitivity.

(b) T—A Mantoux test looks for type IV hypersensitivity against mycobacterium.

(c) T—Allergic rhinitis is a type I reaction.

(d) T—Graves' disease is a type II reaction where antibodies stimulate thyroid cell surface TSH receptors.

(e) F—Rheumatoid arthritis is a hypersensitivity reaction. Osteoarthritis is believed to be a degenerative condition.

36. (a) F—Acetaminophen is not a good anti-inflammatory.

(b) F—Steroids can be given orally or topically as well as intravenously.

(c) F—NSAIDs inhibit cyclo-oxygenase.

(d) T—Anti-TNF-α is a new type of anti-inflammatory drug.

(e) T—Adverse effects of NSAIDs include nephrotoxicity, bronchospasm, and gastrointestinal upset.

37. (a) T—Allergies are type I immediate reactions. They can become chronic, in which case, IgE is still involved.

(b) T—In asthma, airway obstruction can be reversed by 15% or more.

(c) T—Pollen and dust mites are common allergens.

(d) T—Atopic conditions include hay fever, asthma, and atopic eczema.

(e) F—Anaphylaxis is associated with hypotension and shock.

38. (a) T—Densensitization consists of controlled exposure to graded doses of allergen.

(b) F—Antihistamines control the symptoms of allergy but do not cure them.

(c) T—Steroids are commonly used in asthma and eczema.

(d) T—Intramuscular or intravenous adrenaline is important for the resuscitation of patients with anaphylaxis.

(e) T—Many asthmatics can become symptom free by using prophylactic treatment.

39. (a) T—Central tolerance in the bone marrow or thymus deletes the most self-reactive lymphocytes.

(b) T—Anergic cells do not respond to antigen.

(c) F—Molecular mimicry can initiate autoimmunity by breaking self-tolerance.

(d) T—Immune privileged sites can express Fas ligand, causing T cells to apoptose and thereby preventing exposure to sequestered antigen.

(e) T—Regulatory T cells are important for peripheral tolerance.

40. (a) F—SLE is systemic.

(b) F—SLE occurs nine times more commonly in women than men.

(c) T—SLE patients produce antibodies which react with anti–double-stranded DNA or ribonucleoproteins.

(d) F—SLE is associated with HLA-DR2 or DR3.

(e) T—A photosensitive malar "butterfly" rash is common.

41. (a) T—RA is characterized by inflammation of the synovium and destruction of the articular cartilage.

(b) F—Inflammation affects many tissues in RA.

(c) T—New treatment strategies aim to block the effects of TNF.

(d) T—RA occurs in three times as many women as men.

(e) F—The precise autoantigen(s) in RA are not defined.

42. (a) F—25% of people with RA will not be RF-positive.

(b) T—Rheumatoid factor is an autoantibody.

(c) F—Rheumatoid factor is an IgM antibody directed against IgG.

(d) T—Complement activation can occur.

(e) T—Rheumatoid factor amplifies the immune response.

43. (a) F—Reiter's syndrome is a triad of arthritis, conjunctivitis, and urethritis.

(b) T—Hashimoto's thyroiditis is a cause of goitreous hypothyroidism.

(c) T—Myasthenia gravis results from antiacetylcholine receptor antibodies.

(d) T—Graves' disease results from anti-TSH receptor antibodies.

(e) F—Polyarteritis nodosa is an autoimmune disease affecting the vasculature (vasculitis).

44. (a) T—It is a primary deficiency in neutrophil killing.

(b) T—Transient hypogammaglobulinemia of infancy occurs if the production of antibody by infants is delayed or if the baby is born prematurely.

(c) F—Splenectomy is not a cause of primary immunodeficiency but can result in a predisposition to infection.

(d) F—AIDS is a secondary immunodeficiency.

(e) T—Wiskott-Aldrich syndrome produces a primary lymphocyte deficiency.

45. (a) T—Resulting from chronic bronchial infection.

(b) T—Resulting from chronic gastrointestinal tract infection.

(c) F—Rheumatoid arthritis is not associated with antibody deficiency.

(d) F—Antibody deficiency reduces viscosity.

(e) T—Mycoplasma is common in antibody deficiency.

46. (a) T—B cells are polyclonally activated in HIV infection.
(b) T—T cells become defective.
(c) F—Viral replication can be high even during the latent phase of HIV infection.
(d) T—Antibodies are generated against gp120 and gp41, but they are not effective at clearing infection.
(e) T—Lymph nodes become persistently large during HIV infection.

47. (a) T—CMV retinitis occurs at CD4 counts below 50.
(b) T—*Pneumocystis carinii* pneumonia is common if the CD4 count falls below 200.
(c) T—Esophageal candidiasis is common at CD4 counts below 200.
(d) T—*Mycobacterium avium intracellulare* (MAC) is common at CD4 counts below 50.
(e) T—Toxoplasmosis is common at CD4 counts below 200.

48. (a) F—MMR is given at 12–15 months and again at 4–5 years.
(b) F—BCG is not routinely given in the U.S.
(c) T—Influenza vaccine is given to at-risk groups, including those over 65.
(d) T—Tetanus vaccine requires several boosters.

49. (a) T—The Sabin vaccine uses live polio; the Salk vaccine is inactivated polio.
(b) F—Tetanus toxoid is used for vaccination.
(c) T—Rubella is a live vaccine.
(d) F—Hepatitis B vaccine uses surface antigen.

50. (a) F—Hyperacute rejection is rapid because antibodies have been induced prior to transplantation (e.g., by blood transfusion).
(b) F—Acute cellular rejection is mediated by T cells.
(c) F—Preformed antibodies against HLA cause hyperacute rejection.
(d) T—Chronic rejection can be caused by deposition of immune complexes, cell-mediated rejection, or viral infection.
(e) T—The complement and clotting cascades are activated in hyperacute rejection.

51. (a) T—A monozygous twin is genetically identical and should not stimulate the immune system.
(b) T—Steroids are useful anti-inflammatory and immunosuppressive drugs.
(c) T—Antibodies to T cells can reduce the risk of transplant rejection.
(d) F—Most transplants are more successful if HLA molecules and blood group antigens are matched.

52. (a) T—Hematopoiesis starts in the bone marrow prior to birth and does not occur elsewhere unless the bone marrow fails to meet the need for new cells.
(b) T—Bone marrow is found throughout the skeleton.
(c) T—Yellow bone marrow is almost entirely fat.
(d) T—Bone marrow macrophages transfer iron to developing red cells, remove debris from hemopoiesis, and regulate differentiation and maturation of hemopoietic cells.
(e) T—T lymphocyte precursors are formed in the bone marrow but move to the thymus for maturation.

53. (a) F—The spleen is posterior to the stomach on the left side of the body.
(b) T—The red pulp removes old or defective erythrocytes and platelets from the circulation.
(c) F—Most of the B-cell follicles in the spleen will have been stimulated.
(d) T—The spleen starts developing during the fifth week of fetal life.
(e) T—Primary cancers of the spleen are very rare.

54. (a) F—Hematopoietic stem cells are found in the liver and spleen, as well as in the bone marrow.
(b) T—They can differentiate into any of the blood cells.
(c) T—Stem cells self-replicate.
(d) T—Stem cells divide to become lineage-committed stem cells.
(e) T—The actions of growth factors allow lineage commitment and differentiation.

55. (a) F—Polymorphonuclear leukocytes (neutrophils) have a multilobed nucleus.
(b) F—They respond primarily to bacterial infection.
(c) T—They have a granular cytoplasm.
(d) T—They are phagocytic.
(e) T—They are a major constituent of pus.

56. (a) T—Superficial, asymmetric, painless lymphadenopathy is consistent with a diagnosis of non-Hodgkin's lymphoma.
(b) F—Reed-Sternberg cells are pathognomonic of Hodgkin's disease.
(c) T—Fever, night sweats, and weight loss are all features of non-Hodgkin's lymphoma.
(d) T—Non-Hodgkin's lymphoma is associated with inherited disorders such as Fanconi's syndrome.
(e) T—Non-Hodgkin's lymphoma is associated with immunodeficiency (e.g., HIV or immunosuppressive therapy).

57. (a) T—Macrophages are differentiated monocytes found in the tissues.
(b) T—Their primary roles include phagocytosis.
(c) T—They play an important role in the adaptive immune response.
(d) T—They may be infected by HIV.

(e) F—Macrophages are not important in allergic responses (mast cells).

58. (a) T—Chronic lymphocytic leukemia accounts for 20–50% of leukemias.
(b) F—And is a slowly progressing condition.
(c) T—95% are of B-cell origin.
(d) T—Autoimmune hemolytic anemias are common.
(e) F—It never converts to an acute leukemia.

59. (a) T—Acute lymphoblastic leukemia is the most common leukemia in childhood and is rare in adults.
(b) T—The best prognosis is between the ages of 2 and 10.
(c) F—Remission rates of over 70% are seen.
(d) F—80% of cases are of B-cell origin.
(e) T—Etiologic factors include radiation, chemicals, Down syndrome, and Fanconi's syndrome.

60. (a) F—Acute myeloblastic leukemia is an accumulation of primitive myeloblasts in the bone marrow and peripheral blood.
(b) T—It is associated with hereditary abnormalities such as Down syndrome.
(c) F—It can be due to a variety of chromosomal rearrangements (isochromosome 12p is associated with testicular tumors).
(d) F—Only 15% of those over 60 are cured.
(e) T—Patients are often unwell at presentation and can have a bleeding disorder.

61. (a) T—Chronic myeloid leukemia is usually identified in the chronic phase, either incidentally or due to constitutional or leukostatic symptoms.
(b) F—>90% of patients progress to an accelerated phase or blast crisis within 10 years.
(c) T—The Philadelphia chromosome t(9;22) is identified in more than 90% of cases.
(d) T—The Philadelphia chromosome fusion gene product is the target for the tyrosine kinase inhibitor Glivec.
(e) T—Bone marrow transplantation is potentially curative but is not commonly used.

62. (a) F—Monoclonal light chains are produced in a large quantity and are excreted in urine, where they are known as Bence-Jones protein.
(b) T—Neurologic lesions occur due to vertebral collapse.
(c) T—Acquired hypogammaglobulinemia and neutropenia lead to repeated infection.
(d) T—It causes multiple osteolytic bone lesions.
(e) T—Multiple myeloma is a malignant proliferation of plasma cells, which make up more than 10% of bone marrow cells.

63. (a) F—People who are blood group O can have parents who are both group O, although parents who are heterozygous for group A or B can pass on an O allele.
(b) T—Group A people will produce anti-B antibodies.
(c) F—In blood group O, it is the H antigen that is left unchanged.
(d) F—Group AB is the universal recipient and group O the universal donor.
(e) F—Anti-ABO antibodies are IgM leading to intravascular hemolysis.

64. (a) T—Rhesus D incompatibility is a common cause of hemolytic disease of the newborn.
(b) F—It doesn't usually occur in the first child because the mother has not been sensitized to the rhesus D antigen before.
(c) F—Rhesus D is not the only cause of hemolytic disease of the newborn.
(d) T—Passive immunization can prevent the mother producing antibodies.
(e) F—The antibodies are IgG.

65. (a) T—Donor red cells are destroyed by IgM antibodies in the recipient's serum.
(b) T—IgM antibodies can fix complement.
(c) F—Symptoms occur within minutes to hours.
(d) F—Hypotension, not hypertension, occurs, but the other symptoms are present.
(e) T—Release of tissue thromboplastin from lysed red cells can lead to disseminated intravascular coagulation.

Recommended Reading

General Overview

Delves PJ, Roitt IM: The Immune System (Parts 1 & 2). *N Engl J Med* 2000; **343**:37–49 and 108–117.

Innate Immunity

Iwasaki A, Medzhitov R: Toll-Like Receptors Control of the Adaptive Immune System. *Nature Immunol* 2004; **5**:257–263.

Medzhitov R, Janeway C: Innate Immunity. *N Engl J Med* 2000; **343**:338–344.

Walport MJ: Complement (Parts 1 & 2). *N Engl J Med* 2001; **344**:1058–1068 and 1140–1144.

MHC Antigens

Klein J, Sato A: The HLA System (Parts 1 & 2). *N Engl J Med* 2000; **343**:702–709 and 782–786.

Adaptive Immune System

Andeian UH, Mackay CR: T-Cell Function and Migration. *N Engl J Med* 2000; **343**:1020–1034.

Goldman AS: Host Response to Infection. *Pediatr Rev* 2000; **21**:342–349.

Kelly DF, Pollard AJ, Moxon ER: Immunological Memory. *JAMA* 2005; **294**:3019–3023.

Immunodeficiency States

Boxer LA: Neutrophil Abnormalities. *Pediatr Rev* 2003; **24**:52–61.

Buckley RH: Primary Immunodeficiencies Due to Defects in Lymphocytes. *N Engl J Med* 2000; **343**:1313–1324.

Illoh OC: Current Applications of Flow Cytometry in the Diagnosis of Primary Immunodeficiency Diseases. *Arch Pathol Lab Med* 2004; **128**:23–31.

Atopy

Busse WW, LeManske RF: Asthma. *N Engl J Med* 2001; **344**:350–362.

Homberger HA: Diagnosing Allergic Disease in Children. *Arch Pathol Lab Med* 2004; **128**:1028–1031.

Kay AB: Allergy and Allergic Diseases (Parts 1 & 2). *N Engl J Med* 2001; **344**:30–38 and 109–112.

Autoimmunity

Chov EHS, Panayi GS: Cytokine Pathways and Joint Inflammation in Rheumatoid Arthritis. *N Engl J Med* 2001; **344**:907–916.

Davidson A, Diamond B: Autoimmune Diseases. *N Engl J Med* 2001; **345**:340–350.

Kamradt T, Mitchson NR: Tolerance and Autoimmunity. *N Engl J Med* 2001; **344**:655–664.

Kavanaugh A, Tomar R, Reveille J, et al: Guidelines for Clinical Use of Antinuclear Antibody Test and Tests for Specific Autoantibodies to Nuclear Antigens. *Arch Pathol Lab Med* 2000; **124**:71–81.

Knezevic-Maramica I, Kruskall MS: Intravenous Immune Gobulins—An Update for Clinicians. *Transfusion* 2003; **43**:1460–1480.

Weyand CM, Goronzy JJ: Medium and Large Vessel Vasculitis. *N Engl J Med* 2003; **349**:160–169.

Vaccines

Ada G: Vaccines and Vaccination. *N Engl J Med* 2001; **345**:1042–1054.

Transplantation

Halloran PF: Immunosuppressive Drugs for Kidney Transplantation. *N Engl J Med* 2004; **351**:2715–2729.

Pietra BA: Transplantation Immunology 2003—A Simplified Approach. *Pediatr Clin North Am* 2003; **50**:1233–1259.

Poole JA, Claman HN: Immunology of Pregnancy. *Clin Rev Allergy Immunol* 2004; **26**:161–170.

Immunodyscrasia

Chiorazzi N, Rai KR, Ferrarini M: Chronic Lymphocyte Leukemia. *N Engl J Med* 2005; **352**:804–815.

Kuppers R, Klein U, Hansmann ML, Rajewsky K: Cellular Origin of Human B-Cell Lymphomas. *N Engl J Med* 1999; **341**:1520–1529.

Pu CH, Relling MV, Downing JR: Acute Lymphoblastic Leukemia. *N Engl J Med* 2004; **350**:1535–1548.

Neoplasia

Sutton I: Immunology of Paraneoplastic Neurologic Syndromes. *Sci Med* 2003; **9**:274–285.

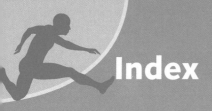

Index

Page numbers for figures are indicated by bold type.

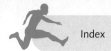

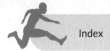

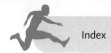

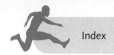

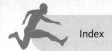